PURGE AND BLEED

Purge and Bleed

PHILADELPHIA'S YELLOW FEVER EPIDEMIC AND
THE STAGNATION OF AMERICAN MEDICINE

Marshall Foletta

UNIVERSITY OF VIRGINIA PRESS
Charlottesville and London

The University of Virginia Press is situated on the traditional lands of the Monacan Nation, and the Commonwealth of Virginia was and is home to many other Indigenous people. We pay our respect to all of them, past and present. We also honor the enslaved African and African American people who built the University of Virginia, and we recognize their descendants. We commit to fostering voices from these communities through our publications and to deepening our collective understanding of their histories and contributions.

University of Virginia Press
© 2025 by the Rector and Visitors of the University of Virginia
All rights reserved
Printed in the United States of America on acid-free paper

First published 2025

1 3 5 7 9 8 6 4 2

LIBRARY OF CONGRESS CATALOGING-IN-PUBLICATION DATA

Names: Foletta, Marshall, author.
Title: Purge and bleed : Philadelphia's yellow fever epidemic and the stagnation of American medicine / Marshall Foletta.
Description: Charlottesville : University of Virginia Press, [2025] | Includes bibliographical references and index.
Identifiers: LCCN 2024054335 (print) | LCCN 2024054336 (ebook) | ISBN 9780813953113 (hardback) | ISBN 9780813953120 (trade paperback) | ISBN 9780813953137 (ebook)
Subjects: LCSH: Yellow fever—Pennsylvania—Philadelphia—History—18th century. | Epidemics—Pennsylvania—Philadelphia—History—18th century. | Public health—United States—History—18th century. | Medicine—United States—History—18th century. | Philadelphia (Pa.)—History.
Classification: LCC RA644.Y4 F67 2025 (print) | LCC RA644.Y4 (ebook) | DDC 616.9/18540097481109033—dc23/eng/20250218
LC record available at https://lccn.loc.gov/2024054335
LC ebook record available at https://lccn.loc.gov/2024054336

Cover art: *A Surgeon Preparing to Let Blood by Cupping, His Apprentice Warming the Cupping Glass,* Jan Baptist Lambrechts, c. 1731. (Wellcome Collection 45018i)
Cover design: Trudi Gershenov

For my wife, my children, and my grandchildren—the keepers of my health

CONTENTS

Introduction 1

1. 1793: An "Awful Visitation" 15

2. Benjamin Rush Gives an Ancient Theory a New Twist 26

3. Philadelphia's Medical Establishment: Divided at the Top and Threatened from Below 45

4. The Fractured Response to the 1793 Epidemic 71

5. America's First Medical Journals and the Battle for Authority 90

6. Cholera and the Emergence of the Gothic in American Medical Culture 117

7. Other Voices: Pharmacists, Thomsonians, and Homeopaths 137

8. Voices Ignored: From Antonie van Leeuwenhoek to Josiah Clark Nott 160

9. After a Century the Mystery Is Solved 194

NOTES 221

BIBLIOGRAPHY 243

INDEX 263

PURGE AND BLEED

Introduction

AMERICANS ENTERED THE TWENTY-FIRST century with a warning that we were on the cusp of a "new age of epidemics." According to epidemiologists, global travel and trade, urbanization, climate change, and rapidly mutating pathogens would combine to produce a series of deadly pandemics. And indeed, SARS in 2002, Ebola in 2014, COVID-19 in 2020, and dengue fever in 2023 seemed to prove these predictions accurate.

Yet despite these warnings, and the epidemics themselves, Americans greeted each disease threat with relative calm—and not without reason. When SARS appeared in China in 2002, the US Centers for Disease Control (CDC) quickly partnered with the World Health Organization to deploy medical personnel all over the world, and as a result fewer than a thousand people died worldwide before the virus was fully contained in 2004. In the United States, there were only eight documented cases—and none was fatal. And when news that a Liberian national traveling to Texas had tested positive for Ebola, the CDC, working in concert with US Customs and Border Protection, the Department of Homeland Security, and state and local public health departments quickly contained the virus. The disease, which had infected close to thirty thousand people in West Africa in 2014, killing more than eleven thousand, was brought under control in the United States after infecting only eleven people and killing only two.

COVID-19 would not prove so easily contained. Nonetheless, surveys conducted in the early months revealed that Americans placed considerable confidence in the ability of their public health institutions and in science more generally to meet the challenge. A Pew Research Center study concluded that 73 percent of all Americans had a "mostly positive view" of science and 82 percent were confident that the scientific community would make still more positive contributions in the future. While confidence in other institutions—governmental and educational—had been declining for decades, confidence in science was increasing.[1] Americans were even supportive in these early months of the containment strategies advanced by the CDC and state health agencies to combat COVID. Restrictions on travel, school closings, and suspension of athletic events and other activities were supported by 89–95 percent of those surveyed. About eight in ten believed that the CDC was doing a "good" to "excellent" job handling the public health crisis.[2]

Over the next two years, the public response to COVID would grow more complex—primarily due to its entanglement with political movements and partisan agendas that had little to do with science or public health. But, as the dust settled, there was evidence that *most* Americans remained confident in their public health institutions. It might be too soon to fully gauge the impact of COVID-era controversies on the reputations of agencies like the CDC. But Americans' relaxed response to the newest infectious disease threat to reach our shores may be instructive. As dengue fever cases reached historic highs in South and Central America in 2023, as cases of this mosquito-carrying and sometimes fatal disease were identified in more than three dozen American states, attempts to alert the public to its dangers aroused little response. Despite the persistence in some quarters of a populist-based suspicion of governmental health agencies, most Americans seem to rest easy in their belief that their agencies would yet again provide protection against a novel disease threat.

That is not altogether surprising. This confidence has been shaped not just by the response to previous threats but by the remarkable advances made in medical science over the past century and a half. Since the late nineteenth-century paradigm-shifting discoveries of Louis Pasteur and Robert Koch, a number of deadly diseases from tuberculosis to polio have been essentially eradicated. And in more recent decades, medical science had blazed countless equally inspiring trails—developments in gene therapy now offer a promising path forward in the treatment of sickle cell anemia, a computer-driven artificial pancreas has been introduced to treat diabetes, immunotherapy is proving an effective alternative in the treatment of certain cancers like lymphoma and leukemia—the list goes on.

In other words, Americans now confront a long list of diseases, chronic conditions, injuries, and even pandemic threats with real confidence that their doctors—and the institutions behind them—have answers.

It was a far different nation that received word of a yellow fever outbreak in Philadelphia in 1793. American medicine was not nearly so well established—at best, the science and the profession were in what might be generously labeled a developmental stage. Philadelphia had opened America's first hospital in 1752 and first medical school in 1765. Yet three decades later, only a handful of colleges had followed suit, and only a handful of American physicians were educated at these; most still received their training through apprenticeship. Of the estimated 3,500 medical practitioners at the time of the American Revolution, only 10 percent possessed medical degrees.[3]

These institutional weaknesses contributed to the public's ambivalent perceptions of the profession. Even more responsible were the actual limitations within eighteenth-century medical knowledge. Almost all physicians still embraced some form of humoral theory, a set of ideas developed in antiquity and systematized by Galen, a Greek physician and philosopher, in the second century. Health—both good and bad—was dependent on the status of the four humors—blood, phlegm, black and yellow bile. These, in turn, were linked to a specific organ—the liver, the lungs, the gall bladder, and the spleen, respectively. Good health depended on the proper balancing of these humors; illness resulted from their imbalance. The basic task for physicians in treating the sick was to design a course of treatment that would restore the body's humoral balance.[4]

To achieve this balance, most physicians practiced some form of depletion therapy. Bleeding has received the most attention; doctors prescribed it for everything from fevers to hernias. Practices seemed to vary regionally: bleeding was less common in New England than in the mid-Atlantic states. But in every region it was widely practiced. While historians have reached no consensus as to its frequency of use, it is clear that it persisted well into the nineteenth century. And the other depleting therapies with which it was combined enjoyed even longer popularity. Purges and emetics, potions designed to cleanse the gut and clear the intestine, were prescribed routinely, even though the most common, calomel—a mercury-based cocktail—caused patients' gums to swell, their teeth to loosen and rot, and their tongues to turn black.[5]

Modern critics like to sneer at the naïveté that led patients to submit to these counterproductive therapies, but to contemporaries, living in a world without antibiotics or painkillers, these methods were recommended by their "results." They *did* produce a change in the body. Bleeding and purging calmed an excited or delirious patient, a pounding pulse was subdued, a person wracked with pain was temporarily reduced to a more restful state, all suggesting to those desperate for hope that something was being accomplished and that their doctor did indeed have some mastery over the human body.[6]

Yet still, the limitations within this medical theory left most illness incurable—and people knew it. They understood that most diseases could be neither prevented nor cured. Pain was an unavoidable part of life, and death lurked on the unfortunate side of almost every sickness.[7] As a result, when a medical crisis like Philadelphia's appeared, medical "authorities" were not perfectly positioned to respond. And when they spoke, they were just one among many vying for attention within an unmediated public forum. In Philadelphia in 1793, the city's leading doctors, men like Benjamin Rush and Adam Kuhn, and the medical profession collected within the College of Physicians competed for attention alongside laypersons, clergymen, and quacks. Home remedies, wonder drugs, ancient cures, and calls for spiritual reform appeared in print alongside the prescriptions of the city's medical elite. One group of clergy linked the city's suffering to moral and religious collapse. Lax parenting, inattentive masters, and unruly children and servants were cited as proof of Philadelphia's culture of permissiveness. The spread of yellow fever had less to do with contagion than the popularity of circuses, horse exhibitions, and the theater.[8]

Relying on ancient diagnostics and therapies, it is not surprising that the city's physicians did not have an effective answer for yellow fever—or most other diseases. What has been more troubling for many historians is that it was another century before America's medical community—its scientists and practitioners—would make any real headway in unraveling its secrets. And consequently, during the medical crises in between— the cholera epidemic of 1832, the Civil War fought between 1861 and 1865—American physicians responded with much the same analysis and therapeutics as those employed in 1793.

Many historians have turned their surprise—even disappointment— into a direct attack on American medicine and its limited imagination. This instinct to find fault, even scapegoat, found a favorite target in Benjamin Rush. By 1844, when Elisha Bartlett, perhaps America's first medical historian, labeled Rush's entire medical system "utter nonsense and unqualified absurdity," it had become something of a truism that Rush's popular therapeutic response to the epidemic—vigorous purging and bleeding—had killed far more than it saved.[9]

Despite this scapegoating and despite the disappointment, no one has mounted a comprehensive explanation for Rush's persisting influence and, more broadly, the failure of American medicine to move beyond a set of dated ideas for almost a century. Some historians have linked it to institutional weakness, the immaturity of American educational and scientific institutions; some have tied it to the theoretical chaos in a medical marketplace unregulated by state or federal governments; still others have suggested that the Civil War impeded medical progress. Some historians have argued that individuals did make important scientific strides, but these failed to find their way into common medical practice—that, in effect, there was a gap between the discoveries of individual researchers and "the practice of the average physician." And yet others have simply asserted that it was symptomatic of Western medicine, an unfortunate characteristic of the early nineteenth century, a period of scientific sterility in some way explained, and even oddly justified, by the extraordinary breakthroughs in the century's final decades.[10]

This last position in particular is not very satisfying. It is not just that the best history focuses on the particulars of time, place, and participants, but that while European ideas certainly maintained some influence, Americans were quickly moving beyond a colonial submission to this intellectual inheritance. To suggest that American physicians and scientists were simply swept up in the general malaise surrounding disease theory ignores the extent to which Americans were intently focused on asserting their intellectual autonomy and making their own distinctive contributions in the wake of—and in the spirit of—the Revolution.

Thomas Jefferson bristled at the accusation of the Comte de Buffon, a French zoologist, that the animals of the New World were smaller and less abundant than those found in Europe. Embedded within a larger theory of East-to-West environmental degeneration, Buffon's suggestion that among America's wild animals there were "very few ferocious and none formidable" infuriated Jefferson. His rebuttal moved from a vigorous defense of American flora and fauna to a critique of the Old World ideas and institutions plaguing his country—and he offered an especially sharp criticism of the medical ideas passed across the Atlantic. This general body of knowledge reflected "total ignorance," and Europeans' understanding of disease, rooted as it was in "false knowledge," was "worse than ignorance." In contrast, Jefferson celebrated his compatriots' ability to combat this, as "the American mind is already too much opened" to be influenced by the jaded ideas emanating from Europe.[11]

Benjamin Rush, better grounded in the state of medical science, if perhaps equally susceptible to hyperbole, was more specific in identifying the resources that could lead America to a new set of medical truths. There was untapped potential within the "indigenous medicines" of the North American continent. America's plants, mineral waters, and even insects might offer cures for "some of the diseases which now elude the power of medicine," such as epilepsy and consumption. And there were additional lessons to be drawn from a human resource unique to America: its Indigenous populations. Rush argued that European Americans could learn a great deal about health from Indian behaviors, including their birthing and child-rearing practices, their diet and active lifestyle, and even their marital patterns. In a curiously revealing observation, Rush noted that Indians managed to avoid the "influence of most of those passion which disorder the body." Envy and ambition were held in check by a general equality of power and property. And in believing that romantic love was effeminate, and the demonstration of a "preference for one woman above another" a source of disgrace, young Indian men were able to avoid those "violent or lasting diseases" that plagued their "civilized" peers.[12]

Jefferson and Rush were not alone; they voiced a widely expressed confidence among American physicians and scientists that they were uniquely poised to advance the world's medical knowledge. The young nation's unique resources were ready to be revealed, and its people were ideologically motivated to make these discoveries. Just as "the convulsions of the late revolution" had unleashed a spirit of discovery across every field—ethics, philosophy, government—Rush suggested that as "truth is a unit" the postrevolutionary generation would discover "antidotes to those diseases that are supposed to be incurable."[13]

Despite this optimism and patriotic declaration of intent, historians have found little to praise in physicians' answers to the new nation's first health crisis. And unable to find anything promising or progressive in the medical or scientific response to the fever, they have sought evidence of America's modern trajectory in the social and political achievements prompted by the crisis. Physicians might not have achieved any sort of diagnostic or therapeutic breakthrough but, it has been argued, a new type of civic leader did emerge during the crisis. When the city's old mercantile elite failed to rise to the occasion, businessmen and shopkeepers from "the middle walks of life" stepped up to coordinate emergency services, opening the door to the representatives and values of a more modern, practical, and secular managerial class. In doing so, they established what one historian describes as a "broader paradigm of citizen voluntarism . . . a vision of participatory, cooperative action for the public good" that continues to define American responses to public crises.[14]

Other historians have found portentous hints of the modern city in the sanitation and public works campaigns launched after 1793 in the belief that better drainage and purer water would deter future epidemics. One historian labeled Philadelphia's ambitious and costly new water system one of these "clear harbingers" of America's urban future. Another historian saw a sign of America's future in the critical role played by the *Federal Gazette* newspaper during the crisis. In providing a critical forum for physicians to introduce and debate therapies, and public officials to issues orders and squelch rumors, the *Gazette* foreshadowed the role that newspapers would play "as important construction sites for the building of new forms of public community in the modern, impersonal metropolis."[15]

Yet another historian added a different wrinkle to this idea that the epidemic accelerated modernizing impulses by suggesting that the crisis played a critical part in the formation of Philadelphia's Black community. When African American leaders encouraged community members to provide nursing care and other assistance in the mistaken belief—spread by Rush and others—that Blacks were immune to the disease, and were subsequently met with more criticism than gratitude, they complained that these attacks provided fodder to persons who "begrudge us the liberty we enjoy and are glad to hear of any complaints against our color." Within this complaint we can see the "first African American polemic in which black leaders sought to articulate black community anger."[16]

There is a great deal of truth in all of these analyses. The epidemic did lead to the expansion of urban services and it did inspire public health campaigns, including calls for urban sanitation. Believing that the disease was spawned in the soggy filth of outlying marshes and low-lying, usually poor, dockside neighborhoods, municipal governments set about draining swamps, constructing sewers, cleaning water supplies, and improving the collection of garbage. And new, different voices entered the public arena to lead these efforts. People from the "middling" walks of life asserted themselves in public affairs; African Americans strengthened their collective bonds; and a new type of secular, civic-minded business class gained power.

But within this emphasis on the hints of modernization within this eighteenth-century crisis one senses the need to find something reassuring in the community's response—a counterpoint to the troubling failures with the medical response, some evidence of America's progressive instinct and trajectory, proof of the exceptionalism that continues to define, for some, the American narrative.

Let us be clear: whatever progressive or modernizing tendencies surfaced during the yellow fever crisis of 1793, American disease theory stalled. The crisis itself, far from prompting a thorough reassessment of old ideas about illness, far from inspiring a concerted and collegial effort among scientists and physicians to rethink their ancient beliefs surrounding health and disease, led to partisan squabbles and the entrenchment of these ideas. It is true that in the years immediately following, a few managed to rise above the professional infighting of the epidemic years while working to decode the nature of the disease and its mode of transmission. But they failed to advance the conversation very far. It was a promising, perhaps even inspired moment, but also short-lived. For within a decade, a contingent of physicians and publishers set about to codify the ancient wisdom—to remove all doubt that this centuries-old analysis represented the consensus within the profession. Over the next few decades, a set of ideas about disease, circulating since the second century, became even more firmly established at the center of mainstream American medicine. They were dressed up in some new ancillary concepts, but in the essential understanding that disease was rooted in filth, that toxic effluvia emanated from swamps and bogs, that diseases like yellow fever spewed from putrefying animal and vegetable matter, would continue to dominate American disease theory for decades to come.

But it is too simple to blame this failure entirely on the medieval ideas of a few practitioners like Rush, or to dismiss it as a tragic aberration within America's march into the present. The story is far more complex. For while it is possible to identify some critical players in the elaboration and defense of these medical theories, their success in doing so was tied to the fact that so much of this medical philosophy fit so well with beliefs larger than medicine. Rush's understanding of disease found its way to the center of medical orthodoxy because it simply made sense to Americans who held certain beliefs about the nature of God's created order, and the power and reliability of the senses God had given humans to navigate this order, just as Rush's commitment to heroic therapies resonated with larger ideas about individual self-mastery. And this means that those wanting to assign blame for the stagnation of American disease theory must look not just to America's scientists and physicians but to portions of the public who asserted their own ideas about medicine, perhaps even contributing to physicians' embrace of ancient ideas that their better selves might have otherwise rejected.

Among the many lessons this history might offer to our own encounters with infectious disease, perhaps the public's role in this story might seem the most relevant. Despite the confidence most Americans placed in "science" at the beginning of the COVID crisis, by 2021 it was clear that the medical community was not so firmly established that its authority could not, at least temporarily, be challenged by individuals and organizations with their own ambitions and claims to authority. In the embrace of alternative therapies from deworming medicines to blood-cleansing potions, in the widespread opposition to vaccination and simple public health strategies, we have seen how American society retains a populist strain willing to challenge and dismiss the conclusions of the medical establishment. We have seen that public attitudes toward the scientific community can waver; that popular—some might say quack—analyses and therapeutics can rival the prescriptions advanced by even the most reputable medical authorities; and that ambitious persons—political, cultural—can easily speak to and manipulate that populist strain.

That is not to say that resistance to the prescriptions of a medical establishment is a uniquely American behavior. When smallpox struck Montreal in 1885, people violently protested public health measures. When the city council announced compulsory vaccination, a mob stormed and vandalized the offices of the Public Health Committee. And within this resistance, we can find elements that resonate with the American response to the recommendations of established medical authorities—a preference for folk remedies, a degree of skepticism about therapeutic practices that had achieved little in the past. But the resistance in Montreal contained some features unique to the city. For starters, the initial vaccination campaign was tarnished by the discovery that the vaccine supply was contaminated, leading to several cases of erysipelas. In addition, the resistance was dominated by French-Canadian portions of the population, who, for probably good reason, were suspicious of any campaign launched by British authorities.[17]

A more comprehensive, comparative look at the responses to infectious disease within different countries would be useful—but that is not what I offer here. Nor was my interest in Philadelphia's yellow fever epidemic driven by a search for its contemporary lessons. Instead, it originated in some fairly straightforward questions about the 1793 crisis and the controversy that followed. But as I proceeded, these questions grew more complex, and I was forced to look at events both decades before and after to better understand the events of 1793 and their significance. For that reason, this book demands a certain chronological flexibility on the part of the reader.

I begin with a brief overview of the epidemic that terrorized the city in 1793 before exploring the response of Benjamin Rush to the disease and his discovery of a "cure." While even in his own time many challenged his assessment, Rush found many supporters—in part, because the theoretical basis for his "purge and bleed" therapy was rooted in some fairly conventional ideas—but also because they were linked to even more ubiquitous themes in American culture about the reliability of our senses and the importance of self-mastery.

But if Rush's ideas were so conventional, why was the response to them so divided? To answer that question, in the third chapter I take a deep dive into the history of the city's medical establishment. On its surface, the city's medical elite had much to be proud of, including the nation's first hospital and medical school. But beneath that facade lay vicious feuds among its most prominent figures—feuds that began in the 1760s and were exacerbated during the Revolutionary War. Complicating these divisions "at the top" were structural changes in the medical marketplace that undermined the authority of the entire profession and its attempts to establish a monopoly over medical practice.

This contested environment set the stage for the heated, unprofessional, and unscientific response to the outbreak of the disease in 1793. In the fourth chapter I look at the response—both the initial debate launched in the heat of the crisis as well as the more tempered search for answers in the years immediately following. There is some good news in the latter. Many physicians worked diligently to find some common ground amid the partisan bickering, some engaged in a promising, albeit unsophisticated type of clinical research. In other words, there is the hint that further research might have yielded some fresh thinking about health and disease.

But in the fifth chapter on America's first medical journals and the battle for authority, I explore the emergence of the *Medical Repository*—a groundbreaking but ultimately poor forum for the assessment of ideas introduced in the epidemic's aftermath. Launched by Elihu Hubbard Smith, a Rush disciple and poor physician, a person seemingly more interested in carving out a place in American letters than engaging in serious scientific study, his journal worked to entrench one set of ideas rather than support an objective pursuit of real answers. As American medical practice seemed to ossify around these dated ideas, portions of the lay public pushed back, but on closer inspection they resisted less the profession's analyses and therapeutics than its claims to absolute authority.

As a result of this professional inertia and lay resistance, the medical community had nothing new to offer when cholera struck the United States in 1832. This crisis is the focus of the sixth chapter. But beneath the stale assessment and therapeutics lay a striking difference in attitude. As American physicians struggled with this new disease, they voiced a helplessness that was not evident in 1793. Contrary to Rush's belief that American physicians were on the edge of eliminating all disease, these newer doctors suggested that disease and its secrets might be beyond the capacity of the human mind to unravel. Amid these confessions, we can detect hints from the public of a gothic-like fatalism about disease—a hopeless assessment of the current epidemic and the medical community's ability to combat it.

While the medical establishment struggled to think its way to a new theory of disease and its treatments, practitioners on the edges of the profession pursued their own explorations. I examine a few of these "other voices" emerging during the 1820s in chapter 7. There is something redeeming in the efforts of pharmacists, Thomsonians, and homeopaths to rethink conventional ideas, and more than a hint of realism in their recognition that the ideas and interests of an assertive public had to be incorporated into their alternative medical programs. But I make clear that none of these offered a comprehensive theory of disease or therapeutics that could be labeled modern, and none provided the sort of direction needed to move medicine to a new paradigm.

More suggestively, in the eighth chapter I take a sustained look at the southern physician who during the 1850s was on the right track in unraveling the mysteries of yellow fever, and possibly disease more broadly.

Josiah Clark Nott was a controversial figure in his own time, and his defense of the polygenetic ideas that formed a "scientific" defense of slavery make him a heavily criticized figure in our own. But his suggestion that yellow fever's spread mimicked the behavior of insects, and his conclusion that these tiny organisms must play some role in its dissemination, represented a promising, albeit neglected direction for medical science. I explore his theories and also attempt to explain how his progressive insights on disease and his archaic views on race sprang not from competing elements in his thought but issued instead from an integrated understanding of biology and history—a fact that points to the troubling contradictions that often challenge intellectual historians.

In a final chapter I take a brief look at medical practice during the Civil War. Much remained the same, but there is also evidence that at least a portion of the military medical service used the extensive clinical opportunities within the crisis to ask new questions. These did not go far, and no new comprehensive disease theory arose to replace the old, but the scientific environment was that much better prepared for the new ideas that would come from Europe in the 1870s. In this chapter I also bring the yellow fever story to its conclusion with a brief look at the late nineteenth-century research that led to the uncovering of the mosquito vector and consequently the rapid elimination of yellow fever as an epidemic threat.

It might seem hard to understand why disease theory advanced so slowly during the century—perhaps even harder to understand why it took so long to recognize the role of the mosquito in the transmission of yellow fever. The historical record includes frustrating references to the annoying insects but only to lament the way their ubiquity added to the suffering of the sick. But these references, like other "why-didn't-they" observations, do not get us very close to the real story of yellow fever in the nineteenth century. For that, we need to look more closely at the people and events, the physicians and the people they served, the researchers and the journals that published and reviewed their work—the historical actors that did command attention, not the tiny bugs that did not.

1

1793

AN "AWFUL VISITATION"

IN 1793, YELLOW FEVER swept through Philadelphia, forcing half of its fifty thousand citizens into flight and killing about a fifth of those who remained behind. For almost two months, the normal activities of America's most vibrant and cosmopolitan city came to a halt. Businesses closed, civic functions were suspended, and once bustling docks shut down. The US Congress, meeting in Congress Hall, extended its recess. President George Washington, after bravely enduring the epidemic's first weeks, took off for the healthier swamps of the Chesapeake.

The city had experienced yellow fever before, but a half-dozen people died before physicians, led by Benjamin Rush, identified the cause as something more than a common bilious fever. It was the death of Catherine LeMaigre, wife of a Water Street merchant, on 19 August that suggested to Rush a more sinister fever had attacked the city. But once he voiced his conclusion, fear spread quickly. Some physicians denied it—Rush had been accused of stirring self-serving controversies before—but the city's mayor, Matthew Clarkson, was disturbed enough to order the city's streets and docks cleaned and to summon a Sunday afternoon meeting of the College of Physicians. Yet when it met on 25 August, this association of the city's most prominent medical authorities failed to reach a consensus. Some were not yet convinced that yellow fever had arrived, and those who believed that it had differed on the cause. While agreeing that, for the moment, the disease was contained to the streets lining the docks, they debated whether it had been brought to America by Haitian refugees or spawned in Philadelphia's own waterside filth.[1]

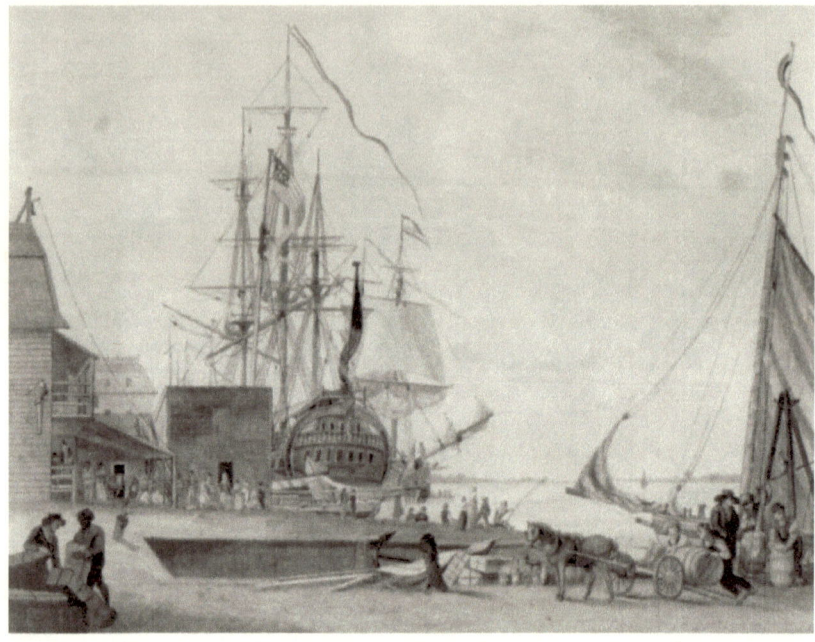

Whether imported by Haitian refugees or caused by the mound of coffee rotting on Ball's Wharf, all traced the epidemic to Philadelphia's waterfront. *Arch Street Ferry, Philadelphia,* engraving by William Birch & Sons, 1800. (Library of Congress, https://www.loc.gov/item/2002718866/)

As Philadelphia's medical experts argued, the death count rose—twelve on 25 August, the Sunday they met, and another seventeen on Monday. By this point, many Philadelphians had begun to take flight, and they continued to flee as their doctors' standard therapies proved impotent. But on 2 September, Rush announced that he had discovered a cure. Drawing from an account of a 1741 epidemic, he urged at the first sign of illness an aggressive purging with jalap and calomel, followed by heavy bleeding—eight to ten ounces on the first occasion, then up to twenty ounces at regular intervals thereafter until health was restored.[2]

Rush's recommendations set off a public dispute among doctors and laypersons that would last well beyond the epidemic. But while they argued, Mayor Clarkson organized a public response of a different sort. On 12 September he called for volunteers to gather at City Hall to draw up a roster of emergency services. With many local officials having already fled to healthier regions, a number of merchants, artisans, and shopkeepers assumed management of the ad-hoc committees that formed over the next few weeks. These committees distributed food, cared for the recently orphaned, and collected and buried the dead. Perhaps the most important of these committees established a temporary hospital in a vacant mansion on the edge of the city. Soon under the direction of merchant Stephen Girard, "Bush Hill" provided care for the poor and abandoned sick, eventually with considerable success.[3]

Yet even after Girard brought some order to the hospital, most of the sick chose to remain at home—and for understandable reasons. In the hospital's first weeks, a trip to the hospital promised certain death, leading many to hide from the carts prowling the city in search of the sick. To provide for private care, caregivers were recruited from among the city's free Black population. Erroneously believing that Blacks were immune to the disease, Rush and other civic leaders appealed to Black ministers and civic leaders to organize their community. Absalom Jones and Richard Allen agreed to help, inspiring a widespread effort that ultimately earned as much criticism as appreciation.[4]

Through September, the fever took a deadly toll—and as the disease spread, so too did rumors of other dangers. Elizabeth Drinker heard that several hundred sick Irish had been dumped at the city's docks, several hundred French soldiers were currently marching from New York to Philadelphia, and five Africans had just been apprehended poisoning the city's water supply. Physicians and officials, armed with more optimism than facts, tried to calm the public's nerves with reports that the disease was abating. Hopes were also fanned by the belief that fall rains and cooler weather would eventually cleanse the city of the toxic contagion.[5] But week after week, the death count rose. With businesses closed, roughly half the population in exile, and those remaining behind afraid to risk infection by walking the streets, Philadelphia was a ghost town. During the last week of September, five weeks after the first documented death, yellow fever claimed just under 100 people daily. On 9 October, the death count passed the century mark; on 11 October, 119 persons died. The following day, a Sunday, heavy rains muffled the sounds of the death carts collecting the 104 people who died. On Wednesday, the 15th, the rains returned—and though the public's reasoning was flawed, the rain and cooler weather that followed did bring relief. Within a week, the death count was cut almost in half. On Sunday, 27 October, only thirteen people died from the fever. And though the disease would claim a handful of victims in the days that followed, Philadelphia's yellow fever nightmare was over.[6]

An estimated five thousand people died during the two-month epidemic—10 percent of the city's population, 20 percent of those who did not flee. Yet, ironically, Philadelphia had been better prepared for a health crisis of this sort than any other American town. The city boasted one of the few medical schools in the country, as well as the nation's first hospital. There were close to eighty physicians practicing in the city, and the most prominent, seeking to provide coherence and authority to local medical practice, had collected within the College of Physicians, modeled after Britain's Royal College of Physicians. For decades city officials had pursued sanitation campaigns to rid the town of the foul water and putrefying debris they believed responsible for disease. They had also established health care services for the poor, including free smallpox inoculation and midwife services. Yet clearly, even this most prepared of American cities was not ready for yellow fever.[7]

We now know that yellow fever is a virus carried from person to person by mosquitoes and that the disease follows a fairly predictable course. From three to six days after being bitten, a victim will begin to experience symptoms: fever, chills, aching muscles, nausea, and headaches. The symptoms will intensify over the first few days—the fever might reach 104 degrees, vomiting will increase. But around day three, these symptoms generally subside. For the lucky ones, this signals the start of recovery. But for the less fortunate, this brief respite only precedes a more ghastly attack—black vomit and explosive bowels, severe dehydration and a parched throat, intense pain in the head and abdomen. At this point, the virus has most likely attacked the liver,

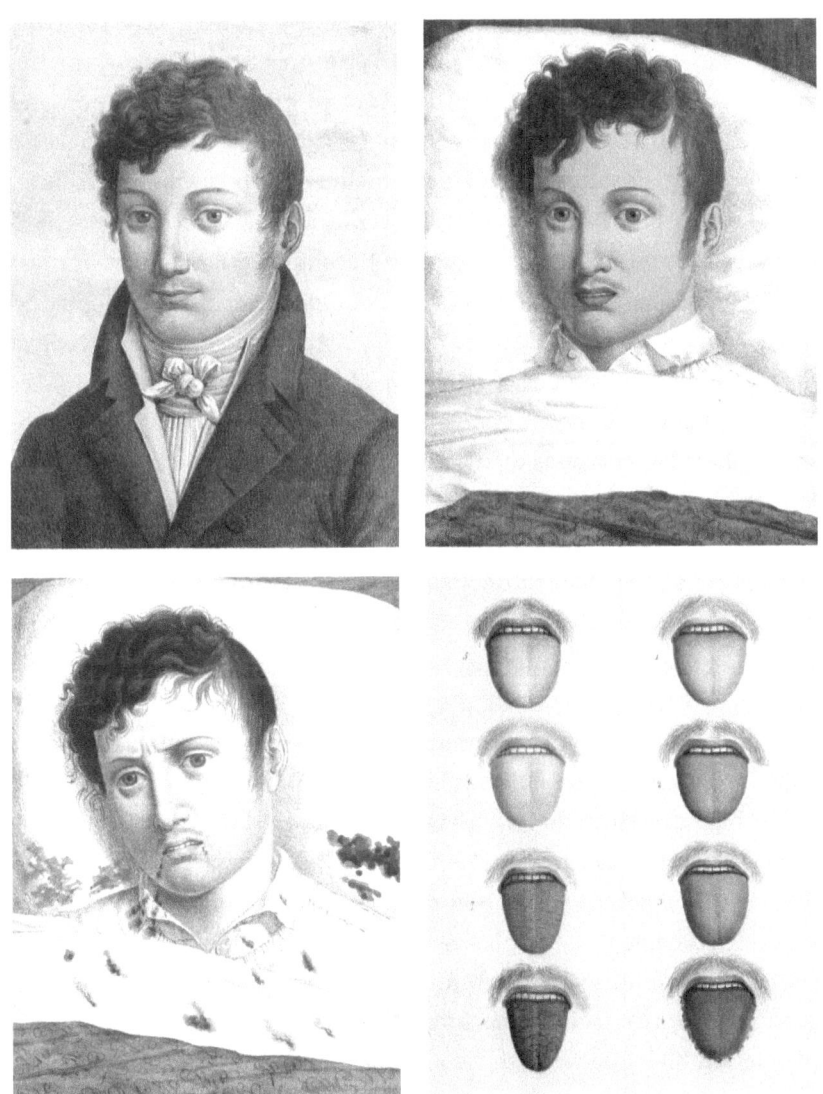

Yellow fever's recognizable and terrifying symptoms. *Observations sur la fièvre jaune, faites à Cadix, en 1819 par MM. Pariset et Mazet . . . et rédigées par Pariset* (Paris: Audot, 1820). (Wellcome Collection)

leading to jaundice, and the kidneys, threatening renal failure. The virus also inhibits the synthesis of vitamin K, and with their blood clotting capabilities compromised, victims bleed profusely from the nose, mouth, and eyes. As victims' condition deteriorates, they suffer delirium and seizures. Death most commonly occurs around day ten from liver or kidney failure, or sometimes an infection linked to bone marrow failure.

We also now know that in previous centuries yellow fever represented more than a deadly scourge: the disease played a crucial role in the contest between European powers for territories in the Western Hemisphere.

Historians have documented the devastating impact of European disease on the Indigenous populations of the Western Hemisphere. Estimates of pre-Columbian populations vary dramatically, yet some demographers argue that as many as 100 million Amerindians lived on the two continents in 1492 with only 10 percent of that number surviving to 1650. Smallpox and measles were the most deadly agents, with mortality rates often higher than those associated with Europe's bubonic plague. These catastrophic rates may be explained by the fact that these were "virgin soil" epidemics—introduced to a people with no prior exposure to a particular disease, thus making entire villages susceptible to infection. Moreover, with no cohort of immunes able to provide care, the sick were vulnerable to secondary illnesses like pneumonia and dysentery.[8]

Yet high mortality may also have been tied to the remarkably homogeneous genetic makeup of Amerindians. Most scholars agree that the Americas' Indigenous population reached the northern continent via an ice bridge linking Asia and Alaska. While there is evidence of "ephemeral contacts" by other migrants from South Asia, Australia, Polynesia, and even Europe, these did not markedly shape the spreading Amerindian population biologically. With no significant infusion of other people to diversify the gene pool, they had far more in common with one another biologically than more genetically diverse Europeans. That is significant as immunologists have revealed that viruses are especially virulent when passed between family members, that is, people with genetically similar immune systems. As patient zero's immune system battles a disease, the attacking virus or bacteria adapts and becomes stronger, so that when it is passed to the next host, it is better equipped to deal with and defeat a similar immune system.[9]

Of course, colonial practices, including wars of conquest, territorial displacement, and enslavement undoubtedly exacerbated the impact of disease and prevented Native recovery. Yet it remains true that the microbes themselves represented an unusually deadly "sword" wielded by European colonizers. But it is also true that as European colonies took root, certain diseases, like yellow fever, acted as a "shield" protecting established settlements against other European invaders.[10]

Yellow fever's potential to actually protect established colonies was a consequence of the environmental transformation that occurred as the British, Spanish, Dutch, and French developed sugar plantations in the West Indies. As these first-generation settlers cut down forests and built small villages, they created nurturing habitats for the yellow fever–carrying mosquito *Aedes aegypti*.[11]

Human populations increased as quickly as the mosquito: the West Indies' total population, which could be counted in the thousands during the seventeenth century, reached over a million by 1750. This was good news for the yellow fever–carrying mosquito as *A. aegypti* is no swamp creature. It prefers the unpolluted, comparatively clean water found in water barrels and buckets—in other words, the variety of water-holding vessels found in populated areas. And this was especially good news for the female mosquitoes, which required ready access to a blood meal to complete the reproductive process. The existence of lots of mosquitoes and lots of humans was crucial to the survival of the yellow fever virus, as the chain of events that enables the virus to survive, much less reach epidemic proportions, is relatively fragile. Only about 60 percent of *A. aegypti* are capable of carrying the disease, and a yellow fever victim's blood is infective for only a few days during their illness. In addition, a female mosquito will seek a blood meal only a handful of times in her life, and as most are essentially unadventurous, not traveling more than a dozen yards from their damp homes, a handful of yellow fever cases will only become an epidemic if there are lots of vectors and lots of nonimmune bodies within close proximity to one another.[12]

As a result, the combination of environmental transformation and massive population growth enabled yellow fever to become endemic to the West Indies and northernmost territories of Central and South America. Sugar planters, and the imperial forces sent to protect these increasingly valuable colonies, could expect to suffer heavy losses upon reaching the New World. But once they did—once a new colony was established and a portion of its residents acquired immunity by surviving one of the regular outbreaks—these now-locals possessed a medical advantage over the next wave of settlers, or invaders, to their region. And the resulting "differential immunity" played a huge part in determining who would resist the disease and thus prevail in an imperial contest. Simply put, this greater immunity allowed the resident populations to defeat—or, more precisely, outlast—the invading forces inevitably devastated by disease. Established colonies, defended by local militia and troops already hit by disease and thus filled with disease-immune soldiers, would stand a better chance against disease neophytes.

While imperial players like Spain, England, the Netherlands, and France understood nothing of the role of the mosquito vector, much less the environmental transformation boosting mosquito populations, they did understand that their colonial adventures had introduced them to entirely new "disease landscapes," and that within these corrupted environments invading forces were at greatest risk of succumbing to the morbid threats. Consequently, the comparative health of their own, longer-established populations provided an advantage. For example, after the defeat of their armada left Spain's navy depleted, they rested the defense of their West Indies holdings on the constructions of fortresses—the most important at the key ports of Cartagena and Havana. Staffed by local militias, disease-hardened troops, and possibly disease-resistant slaves, these fortresses were designed less to permanently hold off an invading force than to delay their advance long enough for the disease to do its work.[13]

While we have gained a deeper understanding of the disease and its historical importance, scholars have not reached consensus on a question central to Philadelphia's epidemic: whether Blacks possessed some degree of inherited immunity or resistance. When Benjamin Rush asked local Black leaders to recruit caregivers from their community, he did so in the belief that Blacks possessed some sort of immunity to the disease. It was a belief first "verified" in America during Charleston's 1699 epidemic, when only one of the recorded deaths was of a Black person. South Carolina physician John Lining gave this belief the imprimatur of medical science in his account of the colony's 1748 epidemic, when he wrote that there "was something very singular in the constitution of the Negroes, which renders them not liable to this fever."[14]

Many contemporary historians identify this assertion of Black immunity and the broader analysis in which it was embedded—that there was something distinctive in the African's physiology—as a catastrophically seminal step in the "medicalizing of Blackness." In the long run, this belief would buttress proslavery arguments that emphasized the peculiar suitability of Africans to slavery—arguments that gained momentum during the eighteenth century as slave labor became increasingly vital to southern rice and tobacco cultivation and West Indian sugar production. Black bodies were inherently more tolerant of the heat and humidity of plantations, it was argued, while white laborers would wilt under the climatic severity.[15]

It apparently did not really matter that this argument was not generally believed by the southern and Caribbean slaveowners themselves. Planters' private correspondence rarely included climate as a rationale for preferring slave labor. Instead, their letters suggested that whites and Blacks, Europeans and Africans, would be similarly tested by Western Hemispheric conditions until they were "seasoned." Yet despite this privately held recognition, the idea of Africans' unique suitability to slavery nicely served certain political objectives, such as challenging the prohibition of slavery in Georgia in the 1740s and defending the international slave trade during debates in the British Parliament at the end of the eighteenth century.[16]

The political value of this belief in inherent racial difference encouraged its survival. Yet since the 1970s historians have argued that there was possibly some basis in fact—that "an innate defense mechanism" might have allowed Blacks to "escape the most virulent form" of yellow fever, and that this resistance might be explained by the fact that these were diseases "their genetic pool had known well in Africa."[17]

The argument is far from resolved. While one side labels the idea of Black resistance "medical heresy" and points out that no genetic marker for yellow fever resistance has been identified as there has been to explain Africans' superior resistance to malaria since the identification of the sickle cell trait, the other side observes that as the disease seems to have been present in West Africa for three thousand years, "it would be astonishing to evolutionary biologists if human populations living in its midst did not evolve some sort of resistance to such a virulent disease."[18]

In other words, for all we have learned about yellow fever, there is much we still do not know. Most fundamentally, we still do not know how to cure the disease. While a vaccine for yellow fever was developed during the mid-twentieth century, we have not yet developed an antidote. As the virus is antigenic, capable of triggering the production of curative antibodies, modern treatment, which consists of alleviating the symptoms, can lead to relatively good survival rates. Yet as access to the vaccine and good care varies, the disease is far from eradicated. The World Health Organization estimates about 200,000 cases occur annually; as many as 60,000 of these are fatal.[19]

Given the persistence to this day of a certain ignorance about the disease, it is not surprising that in 1793, as Philadelphians confronted their medical crisis, they were largely in the dark. They had no understanding of bacteria or viruses in general, much less the specific pathogen causing this disease. Nor did they suspect that mosquitoes were vectors. The agents that we routinely turn to in unraveling some new or mysterious illness were not part of their medical lexicon. Their understanding of health and disease was more graphic, premised on the intuitively logical revelations of what they could see, touch, and smell. Which means, if we really want to understand yellow fever and disease as contemporaries did, we need to set aside our familiarity with germs and contagion and explore it through their eyes—and ears and noses. For in the eighteenth century, yellow fever—and disease more generally—was a sensory experience, filled with distinctive sights, smells, and sounds. Disease was not an attack by invisible micro-organisms, and its cures were not achieved by legions of silent pharmaceuticals. Disease was something you could see, smell, and hear—it was the rosy rash turned oozing pustules of smallpox, the foul-smelling discharge of gangrene, the rusty phlegm and teeth-chattering chills of pneumonia. Disease was detected by the senses, its progress measured by its changing colors and odors. Yellow fever was given its name for a reason, and if we are to understand the terror it brought to Philadelphia in 1793, we need to think a bit less and sniff, look, and listen a bit more.

2

Benjamin Rush Gives an Ancient Theory a New Twist

PHILADELPHIA IN THE SUMMER could be an unpleasant place. Stifling heat forced windows open; horse flies and mosquitoes forced the same windows shut. Privies were too infrequently cleaned, horse dung gathered in the streets, and garbage rotted before scavengers made their rounds. Life in Philadelphia could be hard on the senses. But during the fall of 1793 Philadelphia was a sensory nightmare as yellow fever filled the city's houses and streets with the sights, sounds, and smells of death.

Philadelphians had long known what yellow fever looked like. It drew its name from the discoloring of the skin, a jaundice-related yellowing around the eyes and mouth that we now realize stemmed from the collapse of the liver. But among the sensory indicators confronting patients and physicians in 1793, it was an odor that provided the most useful clue in identifying the source of the illness sweeping the city. Drawing on ancient theories that traced disease to the miasma produced by decomposing vegetation and animal carcasses, Benjamin Rush was certain that the fever flowed from the rotting coffee dumped on Ball's Wharf in July. Now a month later, it filled the air with a putrid smell that hung most thick over the narrow streets crowding the docks.[1] Others believed that the deadly miasma rose from other stinking sources: the garbage that sat festering in the streets, or perhaps the organic bog beneath the houses and warehouses lining the low streets by the river. This muddle of animal carcasses and rotting food, left half buried in soggy ground, emitted a nasty smell that "robbed the air of its vivifying principle."[2]

Whatever its stinking cause, the disease itself produced its own powerful smells and vibrant colors. Bright red blood ran from the nose of the sick, who also suffered through several days of vomiting and exploding bowels. Victims' puke was black and coarse—often likened to coffee grounds. And their excrement, which passed from a green to a deep olive and finally a black color, was so acidic that it burned the rectum and so acrid that it caused people to faint.

To combat the disease, Philadelphians enlisted their own odiferous arsenal. They wore masks soaked in vinegar and camphor to filter the foul air. Others chain-smoked cigars, gnawed on garlic cloves, strung dried frogs around their necks, or tied tar-covered ropes around their waists to fend off the floating toxins. Many kept their fireplaces burning round the clock despite the heat and tossed niter or sulfur onto the flames to add some punch to the disease-killing smoke. The more communal-minded lit bonfires in the streets to burn the death-carrying scum from the air.

Many of the city's physicians scoffed at these unscientific responses, but their own were just as harsh on the senses. Rush urged his patients to take enough jalap and calomel to produce a half-dozen heavy evacuations of black vomit and green excrement. And he drew enough blood—at times as much as forty ounces at a single sitting—to fill buckets with the crimson juice. Rush traveled throughout the city with his lancets, but hundreds came to his home on Walnut Street for treatment. He dumped the gallons of blood drawn daily in his backyard, about two hundred yards from the Bank of the United States housed in Carpenters' Hall.

City officials tried to bring some order to the public's reaction. They issued a decree forbidding street-corner bonfires, but citizens responded by firing guns at regular intervals in the belief that the powder blasts would send cleansing shockwaves. During the first weeks of the epidemic these blasts could be heard over the clattering wheels of wagons carrying refugees from the city—roughly half of the city's fifty thousand people quickly fled the epidemic. But after this initial evacuation, the streets were eerily silent—save for the periodic gunshots and the sound of carts hauling the dead to the city's cemeteries. Businesses closed. The few residents that took to the streets steered clear of neighbors that might in some mysterious way spread the contagion. Even church bells were ordered silent as officials believed their constant tolling to announce the dead unnerved the still living.

Philadelphia's yellow fever epidemic stretched from late August to late October. Between 3,300 and 5,000 people died during this two-month period, perhaps as many as 20 percent of all those who, whether through poverty, foolishness, or sense of duty, did not flee the city. But for those who stayed behind, yellow fever was not an insensible or silent killer. Its presence was evident to all the senses. And as Benjamin Rush argued, this was a good—and logical—thing: "While the cause of the malignant fever is obvious to the sense, it will be easy to guard against it."[3]

Rush had launched his medical practice in Philadelphia in 1769, boasting an impressive education. Like most American physicians, he served a lengthy apprenticeship—close to six years—with Philadelphia doctor John Redman. But unlike most others, Rush had extensive formal academic training as well. He studied anatomy at the College of New Jersey and attended classes in the newly opened medical department of the College of Philadelphia in 1765 and 1766. Even more atypically, Rush traveled to Europe to complete his education. He studied for two years in Edinburgh and then several months in London.[4]

Rush's extensive education did not, however, buy him immediate respect on returning to America. He annoyed established physicians by aggressively promoting the medical theories of his Edinburgh professor William Cullen, which emphasized the nervous system rather than the humors, and portions of the general public by condemning slavery. Rush also complained that his modest family background left him without powerful patrons, and as a Presbyterian, he was the victim of "jealousy or hatred" from Quakers and Episcopalians. Yet despite these sources of opposition—real or imagined—Rush managed to quickly establish a thriving practice and secure the chemistry chair in the medical school. By 1774 he was prominent enough to be at the center of the revolutionary movement. John and Samuel Adams stayed at his home during the first meeting of the Continental Congress. In 1776 he signed the Declaration of Independence. And shortly after the start of the war, he was

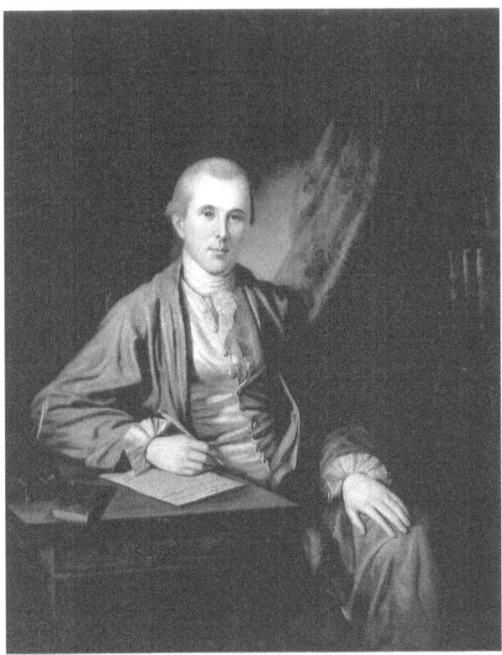

Benjamin Rush, Philadelphia's most prominent and controversial physician, by Charles Willson Peale, 1783–86. (Winterthur Museum, Garden and Library; gift of Mrs. Julia B. Henry)

appointed surgeon general of the Continental Army for the middle states. His tenure, however, was short-lived. Within months he was embroiled in a dispute with the director general of all military hospitals, William Shippen Jr., which ended in Rush's forced resignation.[5]

Rush returned to Philadelphia after the evacuation of the British in 1780 and resumed his practice. He also returned to teaching, and in 1791 began to teach the Institutes of Medicine, a course that since the early eighteenth century had been a foundational piece of European medical education. Herman Boerhaave had introduced the course at the University of Leiden and it was added to the medical school at Edinburgh in 1723. Offering theoretical preparation for later clinical study, the course was incorporated in some fashion in most European medical schools by the end of the century. When the College of Philadelphia's medical school opened in 1765, staffing problems and internal controversies prevented the course from being regularly taught. But after the college merged with the University of Pennsylvania in 1791, the medical school placed the course at the center of its program and asked Rush to teach it. He did from then until 1813. In other words, for more than two decades Rush laid the theoretical foundation for the University of Pennsylvania's medical course of study. A generation of Pennsylvania physicians—at least those with academic training—would enter practice with a background in the theories he taught in this course.[6]

At the heart of Rush's medical theories was a belief that the human body was animated by forces—or stimuli—that coursed through nature. The body was not a self-animating engine, driven by some internal force. Instead, borrowing from Scottish medical theorist John Brown, Rush called it "a forced state," entirely dependent on the stimuli that surrounded the otherwise static human machine. To function—to move and think—humans must be stirred to action by external and internal stimuli.[7]

Rush included light, odor, sound, and air among the "external" stimuli. The influence of some of these was obvious to virtually everyone. Light roused the body from sleep; certain smells could jar the mind back into consciousness after fainting. But other stimuli were more subtle and most people had long lost awareness of their influence. "The current of winds, the passage of insects through the air, and even the growth of vegetables are all attended with an emission of sound," Rush argued. And though we might no longer be conscious of their impact, they still produced "motion in the ear, and through it, upon the whole system." Pure air similarly excited the body's surface (and, in turn, the systems lying beneath) in ways that only newborns could sense. They cried, Rush suggested, because of the "sudden impression of air upon the tender surface of their bodies."[8]

Internal stimuli included food, drink, and blood. And like the external stimuli, these acted in obvious and less obvious ways. For example, food did more than feed the system; the action of chewing stirred muscles in the brain and the heart. And the quantity of food ingested, by "distending the stomach," stimulated "the adjoining irritable and vital parts."[9]

Rush also argued that the faculties of the mind were a sort of secondary stimuli, acting "by reflection" on the body. Like the rest of the body, the mind, including the "understanding" and certain "passions of the mind," was not self-animating but instead must be stirred into action by external stimuli. Here Rush directly rebutted seventeenth-century rationalists like René Descartes and Gottfried Wilhelm Leibniz who suggested that the human mind was infused with innate ideas. Without external impressions, Rush emphasized, humans would be "as destitute of thought as an oak tree." But more tentatively he challenged orthodox religious theorists who generally did not distinguish between the mind and soul; to argue, as Rush did, that the mind depended on sensations received by the body was to suggest that the soul could not exist independent of the body.[10]

For the most part, Rush sidestepped the theological questions surrounding his position yet insisted that the mind was "passive before it becomes active" and that thought and emotion were produced by external stimuli just as "the sound of a bell is the effect of the stroke of a hammer." Moreover, Rush argued that these mental faculties, once forced into action, prompted further responses from the body. For example, thinking promoted circulation of the blood—explaining, Rush said, why "idiots are seldom long lived." Passions like hope and love had a stimulating effect on several of the body's systems, as did emotions such as joy. And, as proof of God's omnipotence, even negative passions and emotions rooted in human sin had been coopted by God to serve God's purpose of promoting human life. Thus malice, lust, and anger could stir the body and its complex systems into healthful operation, albeit more like "the stimulus of a dislocated bone, compared with the gentle action of antagonist muscles stretched over bones and gently moving in their natural sockets."[11]

To receive all these internal and external stimuli, the body was laced with a property Rush initially labeled "irritability" and "sensibility" and later called "excitability." Rush described this as an actual substance found in every muscle fiber as well as the nerves and brain. It served as the medium on which these stimuli produced "excitement," the force or energy responsible for "the vigor or strength of the system." In simplest terms, a stimulus such as light interacted with a substance in the muscles, giving energy or motion to them. More generally, the impressions of the full range of stimuli on the excitability within the body triggered every operation of life—motion, sensation, and even thought.[12]

Rush, a man of science but also religiously orthodox, believed that humans' dependence on stimuli expressed both their integration within the natural world and their dependence on the creator of that world. He also identified a divinely imposed logic within this web of interaction that enabled the body to adapt to the various stages of life. An infant not yet ready for all the sensory input of the world was spared fully developed hearing and sight. Yet while thus somewhat deprived of the aural and visual, the infant found compensatory stimuli through sucking, laughing, and crying. At the other end of life, many of the stimuli that animated the body grew less effective. Eyesight and hearing were weak; lust was diminished. But among the elderly, the body's fluids—urine, sweat, tears—were retained longer and took on a "peculiar acrimony" that stirred the body into motion. Similarly, fecal matter took on a new importance in preserving health; it was retained within the body longer—five or six days—to stimulate various processes necessary to life.[13]

Finally, even though the body was dependent on external sources of stimulation—even though the body was not self-winding—it could generate stimuli of its own to temporarily compensate for a deficiency of external stimuli. During sleep, for example, the body was deprived of many of the stimuli on which it depended, and thus hovered in a necessary restorative but also dangerous state. Sleep was, Rush liked to say, a "tendency to death." But while deprived of the stimulus provided by light, sound, and muscular motion, the body compensated by accumulating urine that served to awaken the body from this dangerous state. More interestingly, dreams, Rush theorized, were part of an elaborate self-defense mechanism through which the body provided critical, sometimes lifesaving stimulus. People in grief, for example, could drift dangerously toward apoplexy while sleeping, but their grief triggered nightmares that quickened the pulse and respiration, thereby stirring the despondent back to life.[14]

From 1791 forward, Rush taught his students that the body was an intricate mechanism driven both to action and thought by stimuli originating primarily outside the body. All of the body's senses—its abilities to see, hear, smell, and feel—were enlisted in the existential work of driving and preserving life. Light, sounds, air, and odors all stirred the body into action by interacting with the "excitability" found in every muscle fiber. Food, drink, blood, and other internal stimuli set in motion a different set of bodily processes. The body was not self-animating nor could it shield itself from the stimuli that bombarded it from every direction; as a result, just as life depended on the sensory forces surrounding the individual, life could be threatened by these sensory forces as well. Health lay in the proper balancing of all these stimuli. When received "collectively and within certain bounds," the individual enjoyed good health. But when a stimulus was received in excess, or some extraordinary stimulus overloaded the delicate web of excitability, the body could be threatened by a surge of excitement—hyper-charged, so to speak, resulting in illness and even death.[15]

John Brown shaped Rush's thinking on this point as well. Brown had insisted that every disease and illness could be traced to either an excess or deficiency of stimulus. With even more singular focus than Rush, he insisted that "the whole phenomena of life, every state and degree of health and disease, are . . . owing to stimulus, and to no other causes." The two diverged on a secondary point: Brown argued that "asthenic" disease—disease caused by insufficient stimulus—was more common. Rush moved toward the conclusion that most fevers were "sthenic," caused by excessive stimulus. But on the more fundamental point—the point that would become critical for Rush in his later battles with contagionists—Brown spoke for both in stressing that all illness could be traced not to "the introduction of foreign matters into the system" but rather to the amount of stimulus received by the body.[16]

This conclusion shaped Rush's understanding of the physician's task in treating illness: restore balance to the system by increasing or decreasing the stimulants that drove it. The calculations could be complex. The physician had to determine whether the disease was sthenic or asthenic, and a familiarity with "all the numerous articles of the Materia Medica" was needed to decide which stimulant or sedative to apply. Moreover, as the passions served as a type of secondary stimulus, the really skilled physician should know how to manipulate these to either boost or diminish the body's excitement. But the principle behind these calculations was simple. As Rush summarized for his students, "the whole secret" of combating disease lay in calculating "in what manner, and in what proportion, we are to diminish, or increase animal life, by the abstraction of natural powers, or by the addition of artificial stimuli to the whole, or particular parts of the body."[17]

Rush was thus intellectually prepared for the disease that struck Philadelphia in 1793. He believed that he understood the body and its relationship to the world. He believed that he understood the stimuli on which the body depended for healthy operation, the role that unbalanced or extraordinary stimuli played in producing illness, as well as the tools available to the physician in combating disease. Yet despite all this preparation, he was slow to recognize the spreading illness as yellow fever. He treated six victims between 5 and 19 August before realizing that something more dire than a common fever was present. But once he realized that yellow fever was in town, his nose led him to the cause—the mountain of rotting coffee sitting on Ball's Wharf. Dumped there on 24 July, this "putrid" coffee emitted the most "noxious effluvia." In a world filled with body-animating sights, sounds, and smells, this rotting coffee was an alien force, a rank miasma that the body could not ignore.[18]

Rush reasoned that this toxic air "acted as a stimulus upon the whole system." It was not disease itself; without a modern sense of viruses or bacteria, he did not believe that the coffee carried or produced any sort of microscopic contagious entity. Instead, he viewed this rank odor as an overpowering stimulus that threatened the intricate operations of the sensory-fed human machine. Resistance was impossible; the miasma was too readily absorbed through the skin, nose, and mouth. In fact, Rush was convinced that virtually all Philadelphians had absorbed the stimulus in the first weeks—you could smell it on their persons, you could even see the yellow tint in their eyes. But unless the opportunistic toxin was assisted by an "exciting cause," the body might neutralize the effects of this stimulus with other stimuli.[19]

The first line of defense was therefore not isolation or quarantine—it was too late for that. Instead, citizens must take steps to prevent the toxin from exciting the systems into a dangerous state. Unfortunately, if the body was "strongly impregnated with the contagion," just a small exciting cause would trigger illness. Heat, fatigue, exercise, intemperance—anything that had a debilitating effect on the body could create the opening the already-present toxin needed to throw the body's systems out of balance. Even sleep was a threat. With many of the body's systems shut down, and with many life-feeding stimuli absent, the body was vulnerable to an overpowering stimulus. Supporting his theory, he observed that most victims took ill while sleeping and reasoned that "the contagion, which floated in the blood" exploited the weakened body at rest by infiltrating the various systems "with such force . . . as to destroy the equilibrium, and thus to excite a fever."[20]

For Rush, it was a frightening but also fascinating situation. And once locked in, his mind ran wild with the therapeutic possibilities. He noted that many caregivers avoided sickness—at least so long as their patients remained alive—and reasoned that hope functioned as a therapeutic stimulus. But after the death of a friend or loved one, an individual became more sensitive to the discordant stimulus filling their bodies. Similarly, he argued, fear was a debilitating stimulus that could open the body to the power of the toxin. But it was all a complicated calculus. If the body was filled with the toxin and consequently overexcited, fear could also function as a depressant, quieting the overheated system. And alcohol, which could debilitate and thus provide an opening for opportunistic toxins, could also stimulate or provoke an "artificial fever" that defended the system from disease.[21]

Struck by the range of exciting causes that could trigger the disease, Rush recommended a preemptive therapy designed to prevent the toxin that coursed through everyone's body from being excited to a dangerous state. He recommended an orderly diet anchored by vegetables and milk. Alcohol and meat should be avoided, as well as overexercise, heat, and emotional overexcitement. In other words, the body's sensory intake should be carefully regulated, its complex systems spared all extraordinary stimuli.[22]

If these preventative measures failed, though, and the invading stimulus produced a dangerous imbalance, Rush had an answer: purge and bleed. A heavy dose of calomel (mercury chloride) and jalap should be taken at the first sign of illness: pain in the head, stomach, or back; chills; or fever. The purgative should be repeated every six hours until five large evacuations were produced. And following these, the patient should be bled, eight to twelve ounces at first, but increased and repeated so long as the symptoms persisted.

Rush was ecstatic in discovering the treatment. When the fever first appeared in Philadelphia, he experimented with several therapies. He gave his patients gentle vomits, applied blisters to their neck and head, and wrapped them in vinegar-soaked blankets. Hypothesizing that the disease was centered in the kidneys, he massaged mercurial ointment into his patients' right side. After consulting with Edward Stevens, a doctor who had dealt with yellow fever in the West Indies, Rush also gave his patients liberal doses of bark—quinine—and prescribed frequent cold baths.[23]

But none of these treatments worked, and their failure left Rush despondent. On 25 August he wrote his wife, Julia, staying safely outside the city, that the disease "mocks in most instances the power of medicine." His efforts, and in fact medicine more generally, seemed defeated. And with science ineffective, he could only pray for the intervention of forces larger than any human effort: the heavy rains and frost that might cleanse the air.[24]

This represented a painful surrender for Rush. He had always argued that physicians should take aggressive action to combat disease. Unlike the increasing number of his colleagues who believed that their role was to gently assist the healing powers of nature, he argued that the "Author of Nature" had only "furnished the body with powers to preserve itself from its natural enemies," not those "bred by the peculiar customs of civilization." In fact, nature could do "mischief" by triggering an incorrect response from the body to certain illnesses. Fortunately, science had enabled humankind to become the "masters of nature," to "arouse, assist, restrain, and control her operations." Yet the first weeks of this epidemic shook Rush's confidence. Unable to dredge from his catalog of treatments a response to the deadly disease, he momentarily abandoned the Enlightenment confidences that had shaped his medical and educational philosophies. In fact, in a letter to Julia he chastised himself for letting these confidences displace the dictates of his orthodox religion: "What powerful antidotes are war and pestilence to pride, vanity, and ambition!"[25]

Rush remained dispirited for days. Letters written just months, even weeks, earlier had voiced his confidence in human progress—the likelihood of abolishing capital punishment and the ultimate resolution of the political turmoil in France. But now he sank into a form of religious fatalism. His own survival, he wrote on 29 August, was "the subject of a miracle." "I fear," he added three days later, "we have seen only the beginning of this awful visitation."[26]

Literally overnight, however, all this changed. While poring over an account of a 1741 yellow fever outbreak in Virginia written by John Mitchell, Rush was struck by the aggressive intervention he prescribed. The doctor had argued that the first course was to purge the gut of the minera deposited by the provoking "putrid miasma" that sat mixing and fermenting with the body's own liquids. Following this, the patient should be bled—and aggressively. "An ill-timed scrupulousness about the weakness of the body," Mitchell warned, "is of bad consequence."[27]

Mitchell's account reminded Rush of the effectiveness with which calomel and jalap had been used during the Revolution to combat various fevers. But his recommendation of aggressive bleeding also resonated philosophically with the heroically minded Rush. His confidence in medical intervention revived, he began to apply the treatment immediately. By 3 September 1793 he was announcing his findings to anyone who would listen, and within days he reported to his wife that his purge-and-bleed treatment was proving 90 percent effective. The disease that just a week earlier had threatened to devastate the city had been reduced to "a common bilious fever." If treated at the first sign—on the first day, even better in the first hour—survival was all but assured.[28]

The discovery filled Rush with "sublime joy," not just for himself and the victims but also for science and his profession. "The conquest of this disease was not the effect of accident, nor of the application of a single remedy," he explained. "It was the triumph of a principle in medicine." He often stressed this point in his letters to the *Federal Gazette*. No longer retreating into religious fatalism, no longer chastising himself for daring to cure the defects of nature, Rush celebrated his and medicine's triumph. And he predicted that this medical victory would lead to others even greater. "I shall give to the world... the history of the rise, progress, persecution, and final efficacy of the new remedies," he waxed. "Properly managed, they might be directed to cure the plague as certainly as the yellow fever."[29]

In just a matter of days, Rush's intellectual and professional crisis had turned into his greatest triumph. Years of medical practice and study converged in this moment of discovery. Not all would join his celebration. Many of his colleagues would question his conclusions, and Rush's dogged defense of his purge-and-bleed therapy would spark a public controversy that continued for years. Following the epidemic, parties on both sides of the debate published works defending their positions—and yellow fever's recurrence over the next several years poured fresh toxin on the controversy. In the short run, Rush found plenty of supporters. His students and medical allies defended his treatment; America's first medical journal, the *Medical Repository,* dedicated several early issues to promoting Rush's medical theories. But in the long run, Rush's reputation was damaged by his part in the epidemic. His treatment was blamed for doing more harm than good, literally killing more than it saved, and his obstinate attachment to a depleting regimen that seemed to fly in the face of common sense made him a villain in many accounts.

Not all analysts were as harsh as nineteenth-century medical historian Elisha Bartlett, who labeled Rush's entire medical system "utter nonsense and unqualified absurdity." More followed the lead of J. H. Powell, whose *Bring Out Your Dead,* first published in 1949, couched its criticism within modest praise. Powell acknowledged Rush's dedication and sacrifice but emphasized that his analysis of the disease and therapeutic recommendations were simply "wrong, disastrously, frightfully wrong." While Rush could not be held responsible for the limitations within the prevailing science, continued Powell, he should have seen the deadly consequences of aggressively bleeding and purging. But blinded by the praise from doctors removed from the scene, heralded as a hero by townspeople desperate for a cure, Rush developed a "pious faith in his own rectitude" that encouraged him to bleed on.[30]

In the seventy years since Powell made this argument, several other scholars have similarly pointed the finger at Rush's ego and personality as much as his flawed science. One argued that Rush was led—and betrayed—by the combination of his temperament and politics. "High strung and combative," Rush blew past many of the "safeguards" within conventional therapeutics. His republican philosophies, moreover, strengthened the appeal of a disease theory that was simple and a therapeutic regimen that common people could actually administer themselves.[31]

A more recent study has tied Rush's uncompromising commitment to his therapies and his readiness to find conspiratorial malice in all those who challenged them to the period's preoccupation with faction. Drawing on Bernard Bailyn's seminal study *The Ideological Origins of the American Revolution*, Thomas Apel describes the radical Whig ideology that informed Americans' thought and behavior throughout the revolutionary period—the exaggerated fear of faction and the hair-trigger suspicion of conspiracy that shaped their responses to British measures in the 1760s and 1770s and influenced James Madison's power-checking strategies in 1789. But even within this context, Rush's paranoia was extreme. He nursed a "near delusional obsession with the supposed intrigues of his opponents," as well as an "overvaluation of his own perspectives." Moreover, Rush coupled these shortcomings to a willingness to find biblical parallels and even inspiration in the trials that accompanied his pursuit of good. With something of a David-complex, Rush celebrated his efforts against the Goliath-like forces arrayed against him. In his battles against individual physicians and the College of Physicians that ultimately sided with his critics, he embraced and enjoyed the role of the "embattled yet righteous underdog."[32]

A few historians have been less critical, or at least more forgiving, arguing that Rush has been unfairly "judged by the standards of modern medicine," and since "he stuck to his conclusions tenaciously, his character and religious attitudes are dissected as possible answers to the riddle."[33] For most, however, Rush and his personality have proven easy targets. Never very likeable, Rush always did have a nose for controversy. As a young Philadelphia physician, officer within the Continental Army medical corps, and medical school faculty member, he was embroiled in one argument after another. Overly sensitive to criticism, coupling an almost morbid sense of professional persecution to an inflated sense of his own importance, Rush could, at times, seem deserving of the harsh portraits. But focusing too narrowly on Rush's character and temperament to explain his medical decisions in 1793 obscures the fact that his assessment of the disease and the therapy he prescribed were entirely consistent with the medical theories that he taught—without controversy—and were rooted, at least in part, in some fairly conventional therapeutic practices.

Rush had taught for some time that since the body was animated by stimuli, and since health and illness were tied to a proper balancing and management of these stimuli, the physician's job in treating illness was to manipulate the stimuli on which the body depended. His purge-and-bleed therapy, in simplest terms, aimed to do exactly that. Purging cleansed the bowels and biliary ducts, dislodging the morbid bile gathered there; it also induced a pore-clearing sweating more thorough than the standard sudorifics. Bleeding, Rush argued, calmed his patients, allowing them to better handle the calomel and jalap. And it opened their bowels so the system-clearing purgative could do its job. Working together, the complementary therapies succeeded in "abstracting excess stimulus" introduced by the putrid miasma and "removing the indirect debility" that characterized an overstimulated system.[34]

Rush's students would also have understood his logic in beginning with a stomach purge. He had taught them that in targeting their therapies they should utilize the natural sympathies that existed between different parts of the body—the stomach and the brain, the liver and the lungs, the intestines and the feet, the uterus and the rectum, the bladder and teeth. By abstracting or adding stimuli to one half of the pair, the "morbid excitement" from the diseased area would be drawn off, diffusing it and rendering it less dangerous. A headache could thus be relieved by inducing a patient to vomit; dislodging intestinal worms would eliminate itching of the nose.[35]

In treating yellow fever, Rush therefore explained that the first course of treatment should be aimed at the stomach. Here he departed a bit from Mitchell, who had argued that the disease's greatest threat was to the abdominal organs—the stomach, intestines, and liver—and should be purged to remove the toxic minera collected there. Rush agreed that the abdomen should be cleared but added that the real danger arose when the disease attacked the brain. Therefore, he purged not just to cleanse the gut but to create an artificial crisis in the stomach that would lure the opportunistic stimulus to an actually healthy organ. "By creating an artificial weak part in the bowels," he explained, he "diverted the force of the fever to them, and thereby saved the liver and brains from fatal or dangerous congestions."[36]

While Rush's rationale for purging drew from his long-held and regularly taught ideas about stimuli and sympathetic body parts, his reasons for bleeding actually drew from generally accepted ideas about fevers.[37] Like many physicians, Rush believed that fever was seated in the blood vessels and that there were two types of fevers: *direct* debilitating fevers that directly sapped the vascular system of "excitement" or strength, and *indirect* debilitating fevers that actually overcharged the system but ultimately weakened it by exhausting it. The former was identified by a weak pulse, the latter by a full or tense pulse. In terms of treatment, the differences were significant. Bleeding was considered counterproductive in treating the former but frequently advised in treating the latter. Rush joined his colleagues in opposing depleting therapies, like bleeding, when dealing with direct debilitating fevers, just as they joined him in encouraging depletion therapy for indirect debilitating fevers. What separated Rush from his opponents was his belief that yellow fever almost always produced an indirect debilitating fever. The victims' full, tense pulse revealed that their vascular system was overcharged, filled with excessive morbid stimulus that should be bled off.

Where Rush more fully separated himself from his critics was in the aggressiveness with which he purged and bled. Even those who conceded that depleting therapies were useful in treating indirect debilitating fevers believed that Rush's prescription of ten grains of calomel and fifteen of jalap every six hours was too severe. And the sheer volume of blood he extracted over a short period of time was simply too much. The body could not tolerate the removal of twenty ounces at a single sitting, they argued, and a doctor should never remove the eighty to one hundred ounces Rush suggested over a series of four or five days.[38]

Rush disagreed, in part because he overestimated by almost double the amount of blood in the human body, but more because aggressive bleeding suited his revitalized confidences in heroic medicine. It was here that he really parted company with many of his Philadelphia colleagues. While a group of physicians led by Adam Kuhn urged a more moderate therapy of quinine and wine, in some cases a mild purge, aimed at alleviating the patient's discomfort while nature did its healing work, Rush scoffed at their cowardice. He would later write that this "undue reliance upon the powers of nature in curing diseases" was impeding the progress of medicine. But in 1793 he was more blunt in declaring that this "superstition" was taking lives. History may have taught that "all new remedies are forced to pass through a fiery ordeal," but this lesson did not temper the fact that this stodgy adherence to a weak-kneed therapy was tantamount to administering "poison to our citizens."[39]

This sort of rhetoric filled the public debate between Rush and his opponents during and after the epidemic. Far from engaging in a scholarly dialogue over etiology and therapy, they accused one another of malpractice and even murder. Rush argued that Kuhn and his followers, by refusing to employ Rush's therapy, were responsible for "desolating three fourths of our city." If nothing else, added Rush, Kuhn should keep his opinions to himself and avoid "adding to the mortality of the disorder." One of Kuhn's surrogates, Thomas Ruston, countered that Rush's aggressive bleeding was as dangerous as clapping "a knife at once to the throat." For the most part, Rush was the first and most ready to escalate the war of words. But in his mind there was simply too much at stake. Embedded as it was within a more comprehensive set of ideas about health and disease, the role of physicians, and medicine's enormous potential to eradicate illness and save human lives, Rush's yellow fever treatment represented all that he stood for as a physician and, perhaps more powerfully, as a teacher.[40]

Just two years earlier Rush had been handed a heady assignment. Asked to teach the Institutes at the medical school, he would be following in the footsteps of some medical giants. Like Herman Boerhaave at Leiden and William Cullen at Edinburgh, Rush laid the theoretical foundation for a generation of physicians. But as he prepared his lectures, he worried that his own medical principles were too derivative. David Ramsay recounted after Rush's death that when he visited the medical school professor in 1789, Rush was in the process of rethinking the overarching theories that guided his work. The system of his mentor, Cullen, "was tottering." In its place, John Brown's theories were pointing Rush toward a "more simple and consistent system of medicine than the world had yet seen." Over the next two years he refined this new system—until it became the basis of what he taught in the Institutes beginning in 1791. But now, just two years later, his theories were under public attack. Unlike the fawning students who recorded his lectures virtually verbatim, other physicians (including other medical school faculty like Kuhn) were publicly challenging him in the press. And so, to the extent that Rush's character did play a part in his rigid defense of his theories, we might look less to an "unquestioning assumption of special providence and superiority," as J. H. Powell argued, than to the anxiety of a teacher threatened with the loss of status and authority which would accompany the rejection of all that he taught.[41]

In the end, Rush's extensive paper trail—his lecture notes, published writings, and correspondence—leave his analysis and prescription, his errors, and perhaps even his motives accessible to analysis. More difficult to assess—yet more important to understanding the significance of all this for American medical history—is the response of the rest of the community: the physicians who rallied to his side; the public who accepted, perhaps even preferred, his therapeutic course; and the physicians who opposed him and his recommendations. Given that Rush's prescriptions were not that far removed from the mainstream, this last question in particular requires a more complex answer than many have provided. The opposition of Rush's peers cannot be read through the lens of later critics or informed by modern understandings of the terrible flaws within Rush's analysis. It must be explored within the context of Philadelphia's medical community in 1793.[42]

To do that we need to take a closer look at the rancor that accompanied this debate. Scientific disagreement is not new; at times it has led to a constructive search for new principles, the beneficial formation of a new synthesis. But in 1793, the medical and scientific community behaved in the most unscientific of ways—with personal invective rather than respectful dialogue, with rigid defense of narrow theories rather than a cooperative search for common ground—and the resulting disharmony not only inhibited constructive collaboration but helped fix certain positions on the edges of the theoretical spectrum.

Ultimately, answering these questions will help us understand not just the 1793 epidemic but its role in the elaboration of American disease theory—why Americans in 1832, during the cholera epidemic, were still thinking about disease in much the same way they had almost a half century earlier. But in order to answer these questions, we need take a step backward in time and look at the personalities and issues shaping Philadelphia's medical community over the previous quarter century. This requires that we look at its leading figures and the elaboration of its institutions, as well as changes within the larger medical marketplace that presented the professional community with both opportunities and challenges.

3

Philadelphia's Medical Establishment

DIVIDED AT THE TOP AND THREATENED FROM BELOW

IN 1793, PHILADELPHIA WAS ostensibly better prepared for a health crisis than any other city in America. It housed the nation's first medical school as well as the nation's oldest hospital. Close to eighty physicians practiced in the city, and almost certainly more of these had formal academic training, including European degrees, than the medical corps of any other American city. To further strengthen the profession, Philadelphia's medical elite had united within a College of Physicians in 1787. Modeled loosely after Britain's Royal College of Physicians, this professional society sought "to advance the science of medicine" and encourage "the advancement of useful knowledge." Beyond the institutional achievements of the city's doctors, Philadelphia city officials had long embraced public health as a civic responsibility. As early as 1762 laws had been passed designed to rid the city of garbage and contaminants. Streets were paved and pitched to encourage runoff; distillers, butchers, soap-boilers, and other tradespeople were fined if they discharged offensive debris in the streets. Portions of the city's open sewer were covered, and the docks were regularly inspected. Officials had even established health care services for the poor, including midwife services and free smallpox inoculations.[1]

But beneath this impressive professional and institutional facade, Philadelphia's medical community was rife with division. Some of its most prominent figures hated one another, and its historic institutions, having been founded in discord rather than cooperation, exercised limited authority among practitioners. Even the College of Physicians was less an ambitious clone of Britain's powerful Royal College than a rather modest attempt to strengthen the profession's status while mending internal wounds and bringing some "order and uniformity"—read civility and cooperation—to Philadelphia medical practice.[2]

As a result, Philadelphia's physicians responded badly to the epidemic in 1793. Rather than presenting a united and authoritative voice, they bickered. Rather than pooling their talents and experience to assess the rapidly accumulating data on the spreading disease, they engaged in a public feud over its origins and treatment. Rather than using this epidemic to strengthen their position within the community, they squandered the opportunity to solidify their status and undermined confidence in medicine and its practitioners.

At the heart of this disharmony lay an old feud involving three of the city's most prominent physicians: John Morgan, William Shippen Jr., and Benjamin Rush. Their biographies might suggest grounds for mutual respect and common vision. Morgan and Shippen, in particular, pursued similar and overlapping paths to Philadelphia medical practice. Separated by only one year in age, they both attended Samuel Finley's prep school in West Nottingham, and after taking their American degrees—Morgan at the College of Philadelphia and Shippen at the College of New Jersey—they both went to Europe to complete their medical educations. Morgan's stint as a regimental surgeon during the French and Indian War allowed Shippen to take this path first in 1758, but Morgan followed two years later, carrying with him letters for his compatriot then studying in London. In fact, with Shippen having just completed his London studies and departing for Edinburgh, Morgan replaced him as a boarder in the home of the famous anatomy instructor John Hunter. Also like Shippen, Morgan joined a social circle of Americans living in the English capital and was mentored by the American expatriate and Quaker physician John Fothergill. How much Shippen and Morgan actually saw one another over the next year is unclear, but Shippen returned to London in 1761 and watched the coronation of George III with his fellow Philadelphian.

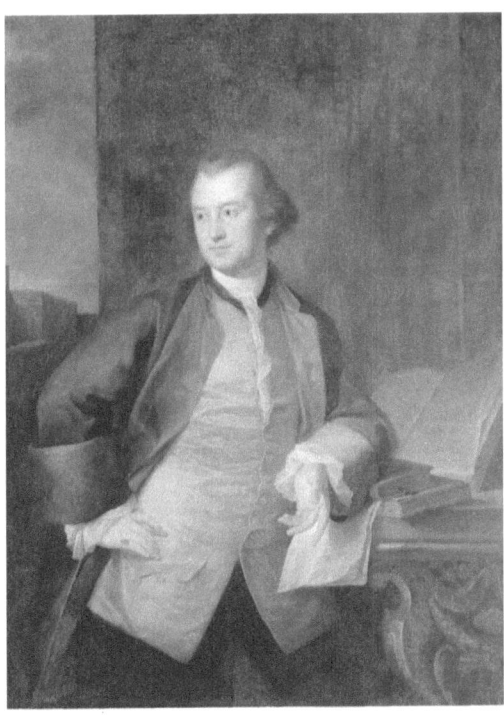

John Morgan, American medical education visionary, by Angelica Kauffmann, 1764. (National Portrait Gallery, Smithsonian Institution; this acquisition was made possible by a generous contribution from the James Smithson Society)

And when Shippen returned to America shortly after, Morgan set off for Edinburgh where he found living quarters in a residence recommended by Shippen.[3]

While neither young physician left much of a written record, it is clear that the two discussed the status of their profession in America and the absence of a medical school that had forced them to complete their educations abroad. And letters from other American students studying abroad reveal that Morgan and Shippen, along with their mentor Fothergill, plotted the solution. In letters to their fathers, both Thomas Ruston and Samuel Bard described the "scheme" being hatched by Shippen and Morgan: they would launch "the first medical college in America" and anchor its faculty. But it is also clear that at some point the visions of the two ambitious doctors diverged. As their European educations unfolded in different ways, their conceptions of the sort of medical school they would establish did as well.[4]

Shippen spent the bulk of his time studying in England where medical training was largely clinical in nature. He walked rounds at St. Thomas's Hospital, and like other British medical students, purchased admission to lectures offered by independent instructors—Shippen studied anatomy with John Hunter and obstetrics with Colin Mackenzie. Shippen also spent a year in Edinburgh where medical training had taken on the academic character that would come to define formal medical education over the next century. There, students pursued a core curriculum that included materia medica, chemistry, medical theory, medical practice, and anatomy.[5] They spent six to seven hours a day in lecture, with rounds within the local infirmary only optional. Shippen stayed in Edinburgh long enough to earn his M.D., but his English experience seems to have been the more formative, and therefore it is not surprising that when he returned to America, he presented his proposal for a new medical school to the manager and treasurer of the Pennsylvania Hospital—not the Trustees of the College of Philadelphia. In his experience, and within his vision, the hospital, not the university, should be the center of a clinically based medical education.[6]

In 1762, however, the Pennsylvania Hospital was not interested in sponsoring a medical school. The hospital was in poor financial shape and not prepared to underwrite Shippen's educational project. Nor could the hospital expect to tap the same sort of social and ecclesiastical institutions that supported British hospitals—they simply did not exist in America. It is also possible that Thomas Bond, one of the hospital's founding physicians, had the final say. Bond had provided informal clinical instruction to medical students for some time and had just arranged to provide a series of formal lectures the following year. This influential member of the hospital staff might have been anxious to protect his educational turf.[7]

After his proposal was rejected, Shippen announced that he would give a series of lectures on anatomy. He also opened a private practice, which by 1765 grew to include obstetrics—still unusual for a male practitioner. By this time, Morgan had completed his studies in Europe and taken a medical version of the Grand Tour. He socialized with the Duke of York, gained an audience with Pope Clement, and discussed politics and

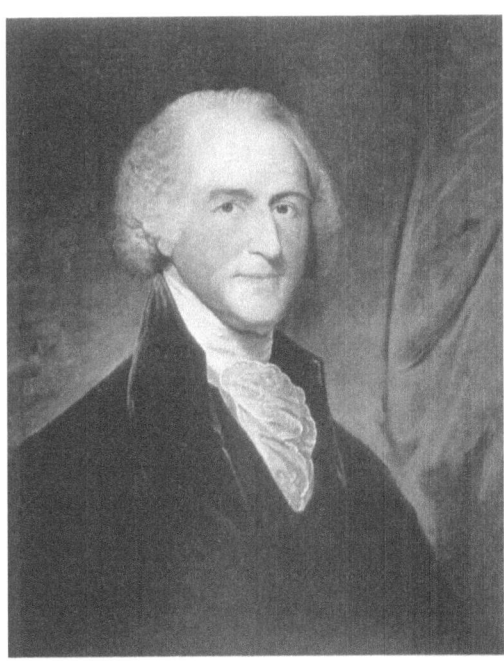

William Shippen Jr., director general of the Continental Army military hospitals, unknown date. (National Library of Medicine)

philosophy with Voltaire and specimen preservation with the Italian pathologist Giovanni Battista Morgagni. The connections Morgan cultivated in his travels paid dividends. He was named a correspondent of France's Royal Academy of Surgeons, and he was admitted to Britain's Royal Society, Britain's Royal College of Physicians, and the Arcadian Belles Lettres Society of Rome.[8]

By the time Morgan returned to Philadelphia in 1765, he boasted an impressive international reputation and considerable academic clout. And his credentials may explain, in part, the more favorable response his proposal for a medical school received. When he presented his ideas to the trustees of the College of Philadelphia—not the Pennsylvania Hospital—they immediately embraced his plans. But it is more likely that he succeeded where Shippen had not for other reasons. For starters, Morgan had carefully cultivated support among influential Pennsylvanians—most critically, two trustees of the college, James Hamilton and Richard Peters, and the colony proprietor, Thomas Penn. As important, the proposal he finetuned during his studies better suited the institutional vision and ego of the college to which he made his appeal.[9]

Morgan spent the bulk of his time in Europe in Edinburgh. He spent a year in London studying with the Hunter brothers, William and John, Britain's preeminent anatomists. Morgan also walked rounds at St. Thomas's, but more academic in nature than Shippen and simply more intellectually curious, Morgan was inspired by Edinburgh's theory-heavy, academic approach to medical training. By the time he returned to America he had drafted a proposal for a medical school that was modeled largely after the Scottish school. Students would take courses in anatomy, materia medica, botany, chemistry, and both medical theory and practice, leading to an M.D. Medical training, in other words, would be centered in the college's classrooms, not the unaffiliated hospital.[10]

Morgan thus arrived with a plan that would place medical education within the College of Philadelphia. Access to the profession and control over what physicians learned—in effect, medical authority—would be situated within the college, not the hospital. Morgan's was a plan that spoke to the institutional ethos of the college—and its trustees embraced his proposal enthusiastically.

Not everyone, however, celebrated the announcement. Shippen was furious. Adding salt to the wound, Morgan did not fully reference Shippen's earlier proposal or their earlier discussions when he introduced the new medical school in a 1765 address, noting only that Shippen had offered "hints of a plan for giving medical lectures." Morgan contrasted this partial plan with his own "full and enlarged plan." In a moment of restrained largesse, Morgan did reach out to Shippen in the address—he suggested that should the trustees decide to appoint Shippen professor of anatomy at his new school, it would be a "circumstance favorable to our wishes." But the gesture was far from enough for Shippen. While accepting the position, he reminded the trustees that he had proposed something similar three years earlier. It was a plan he had "first communicated to Morgan" while in London, he explained, but he had decided to wait until Morgan returned before pursuing it further.[11]

While Shippen steamed, Morgan pressed ahead with his college plans, clearly uninterested in repairing the rift. In fact, just a year later, when Morgan pulled together a group of young physicians to organize a medical society, he did not include Shippen. Shippen and the rest of the Philadelphia medical community were invited to participate, but snubbed as a founder, Shippen refused.

Over the next decade, the feud between Morgan and Shippen may have calmed—but it still simmered. Thomas Bond observed in 1769 that their quarrels were undermining the status of the medical school. The school would not make "a considerable figure," he wrote Benjamin Franklin, until "we straighten one or two crooked ribs amongst us." Nor did the outbreak of revolutionary violence in 1775 inspire the two to reconcile for the sake of the cause. In fact, just the opposite occurred. The medical needs of the American army prompted an even more vicious quarrel between Morgan and Shippen.[12]

Shortly after the Battle of Bunker Hill, the Continental Congress ordered the formation of a general hospital to care for General George Washington's troops. Benjamin Church was named director general and chief physician of the new hospital, but his tenure was brief. Within just months he had been charged with treason and dismissed. John Morgan was named his successor—but support for the Philadelphia doctor was not unanimous. Washington told fellow Virginian Richard Henry Lee that he was sorry Lee's brother-in-law William Shippen Jr. had not been named instead.[13]

Within a year, Morgan may have felt the same, for organizing and overseeing medical care for the embryonic revolutionary army proved an impossible task. The challenges with collecting supplies, recruiting personnel, and equipping facilities were difficult enough. But faced with a weak congress, regional rivalries, and the competing ambitions of local medical providers, Morgan found his job virtually impossible. He immediately found himself at odds with the surgeons staffing the regimental hospitals, who expected Morgan to supply their needs but not interfere with their operations. Morgan, in turn, insisted on raising the qualifications for service in the hospitals—and personally examined many of the regimental surgeons already unhappy with the demanding director general. As a result, the medical service was in disarray well before the disastrous campaign of 1776 flooded the hospitals with sick and wounded.[14]

Morgan's appeals to Congress to clarify the relationship between the regimental and general hospital and the chain of command between Morgan and regimental surgeons drew no effective response. Just the opposite: in July 1776 Congress further complicated the situation by establishing a separate Hospital of the Flying Camp to serve Pennsylvania, New Jersey, and Maryland militia stationed in New Jersey, and named a director—William Shippen Jr.[15]

In the months that followed, while disturbing official reports and even more frightening rumors flowed from Morgan's general hospital, Shippen sent Congress rosy reports of healthy troops and empty hospital beds. The revitalized tensions between the old rivals quickly became a turf war as Shippen petitioned Congress to restrict Morgan's authority to those troops stationed east of the Hudson River. Congress acquiesced, and with Washington's army all but removed from New York, Morgan and his hospital were reduced to minor pieces within the medical service. To add salt to the wound, Shippen also demanded the transfer of all medical supplies still in Morgan's possession. Washington turned this request into an order—and with Morgan's position undermined and reputation largely ruined by the reports of incompetence, Congress dealt the final blow. In January 1777 it dismissed Morgan from service, leaving Shippen de facto head of the American medical service.[16]

But Morgan was not one to withdraw quietly. He immediately mounted a campaign to clear his name and smear the villain who, he believed, had engineered his dismissal. He demanded a hearing before Congress and argued his case through the press. The problems within the medical service could be traced to the maladministration of regimental surgeons, he explained. They falsified returns, encouraged malingerers, and made fraudulent drafts against the general hospital. And when he had attempted to rein in their corrupt practices, they united against him. But even more responsible for the conspiracy against him, he claimed, was William

Shippen. According to Morgan, Shippen aspired to a position in the military hospitals not to serve the nation but rather to secure "a more gentlemanly life," an alternative to "a drudging private practice." And, Morgan added, Shippen had attacked him in a thinly veiled attempt to replace him. He had been driven from office not by any fault of his own but rather by the machinations of a man who lacked "the virtue to imitate . . . (but would still) rise to his envied position."[17]

In June 1779 Morgan succeeded in the first of his objectives. A congressional committee charged with investigating Morgan's complaints concluded that the disgruntled former director general had "vindicated his conduct in every respect." By this point, however, Morgan was more fully engaged in bringing down the man who had replaced him. And he was joined in this effort by Benjamin Rush.[18]

Rush was a bit younger than Shippen and Morgan, but his path to medicine was similar. Like the other two, he attended Samuel Finley's school in West Nottingham before enrolling, like Shippen, at the College of New Jersey in 1759. Following graduation, he served a six-year medical apprenticeship under John Redman in Philadelphia, as had Morgan. During this time, Rush was among the ten students enrolled in Shippen's first set of private anatomy lectures in 1762. And after the College of Philadelphia opened its medical school in 1765, Rush attended classes taught by Morgan and Shippen. He traveled to Europe to complete his medical education in 1766, studying for two years and taking his degree at Edinburgh, and just over six months in London, making rounds at St. Thomas's and Middlesex Hospitals and studying anatomy with John Hunter.[19]

An ardent Whig and signer of the Declaration of Independence, Rush was named surgeon general for the Middle Department in 1777, a position that placed him under the authority of Director General William Shippen. Rush assumed the position in April, and by October he was complaining about the condition and organization of the military hospitals. In letters to John Adams, Nathanael Greene, William Duer, and ultimately George Washington, Rush described the woeful shortage of supplies and crowded conditions in the hospitals. The sick and injured were poorly attended and just as poorly disciplined. All sorts of irregularities—especially drunkenness—resulted. And consequently, if the injured did manage to survive their hospital stays, they returned to the ranks ill-suited for duty. "The discipline of a whole year is lost in one month," he complained, "by the total neglect of it which prevails in our hospitals."[20]

For the most part, Rush blamed the structure of the medical service, more specifically the concentration of too many responsibilities in the office of the director general. The failure to separate the business of purveyance from the medical duties of treatment was a particular problem, providing medical department officers "unlimited opportunities to defraud the public." But on occasion, Rush let down his guard and directed his criticism at Shippen, who, Rush charged, turned a blind eye and at times actually joined in the profiteering and peculation within the medical office. "He is both ignorant and negligent of his duty," Rush wrote Adams.[21]

In December Rush urged Duer to convey his concerns to Congress. By this time, Shippen was well aware of the activities of his disgruntled subordinate and characterized Rush's complaints as part of a campaign to replace him. Rush insisted that he aimed only to reform the medical department and would resign to demonstrate his intention. When he was subsequently asked to appear along with Shippen before a congressional committee, Congress called his bluff. New Jersey delegate John Witherspoon suggested that one of the two combating physicians needed to resign, and since Rush had several enemies in Congress, it should be him.[22]

Rush left the medical service in January 1778—and the gloves came off. He wrote General Washington of hospital stores being siphoned off by high-ranking officials and of meat and game being purchased at the director general's request that never found their way to the sick and injured. He described the overcrowded hospital conditions that bred disease and Shippen's callous indifference. "The Director General," he reported, "never entered the hospital but once during about six weeks' residence in the village of Bethlehem, although the utmost distress and mortality prevailed in the hospital at that time." To Nathanael Greene he accused Shippen of lying about the number of hospital fatalities. "I was deceived," Rush wrote, "by counting the number of coffins that were daily put in the ground." To Daniel Roberdeau Rush offered his most bitter assessment of Shippen's character—a "man who had been absorbed for the last 15 years of his life wholly in pleasure . . . whole nights and days in reveling and debauchery." And he followed with a more loaded set of questions: "What would be the fate of a general officer who would throw away the fate of 1000 Continental troops in a drunken frolic or sell them to an enemy? He would expiate his crime with his life. And shall 1000 of your brave soldiers be lost ignobly in a hospital? Shall the cry of murder resound through every graveyard in the villages of Pennsylvania?"[23]

Rush thus had plenty to offer when John Morgan reached out to him in 1779 about his experience under Shippen. By now Rush estimated that "many thousands of our brave countrymen" had died under the maladministration of Shippen, and he pledged to support Morgan's efforts in "fixing the guilt of neglecting and robbing our hospitals upon the person who has done both." Working together, the two built an elaborate case alleging that Shippen had misappropriated resources, profiteered through speculating in hospital stores, and demonstrated a crass disregard for the wounded and sick placed in his care. And Congress found the allegations credible enough to order a court martial of the director general. Immediately, Morgan set off on a journey throughout the Northeast to secure depositions from soldiers and hospital staff familiar with Shippen and the hospitals he managed. And armed with these, Morgan led the prosecution.[24]

Yet despite the evidence mustered by Morgan and Rush, in July 1780, after a five-month trial, Shippen was acquitted on all charges. The court did admonish him for engaging in "reprehensible" speculation. But for Morgan, this reprimand fell far short of the public stoning he believed Shippen deserved. So, for the next four months, Morgan waged a relentless campaign in the press against his old rival.[25]

The depositions that Morgan had collected for the trial were now summarized and excerpted in the pages of the *Pennsylvania Packet* in an extended "Appeal to the Free Citizens of the United States." The public heard from tavernkeepers who swore that Shippen sold them goods from the hospital's supply of wine and sugar, from wagon owners who complained that their wagons were pressed into Shippen's private commercial service, and from a bookkeeper who claimed that Shippen had asked him to alter books to cover up Shippen's misdeeds. Camp visitors testified that

Shippen's hospital grounds were covered "with excrement and nastiness" and wards were overcrowded and poorly ventilated. Injured soldiers lay for days untreated, their blood-soaked shirts eventually drying hard to their wounds. And while an estimated hundreds died from neglect, Shippen and his staff, according to one innkeeper, "lived in riot, caroused nightly, and HAD LIQUORS BROUGHT TO THEM IN BUCKETS FULL FROM THE HOSPITAL STORES."[26]

Depositions taken from hospital physicians were also laid before the public. Dr William Brown swore that the unsanitary conditions led to the spread of "malignant diseases." Dr. James Tilton stated that due to "neglect in the directorial branch of the hospital," soldiers "suffered and died in a manner that was truly shocking to humanity."[27]

For two months Morgan landed blow after unanswered blow. But in November, Shippen took his case to the press. In the same pages of the *Pennsylvania Packet* he defended his conduct and reduced Morgan's attacks to "the malice of a displaced and angry man." But his defense lacked the power of Morgan's. Shippen relied primarily on repeated reminders that he had been acquitted. And as for the "reprehensible speculation" for which he had been reprimanded, he stressed that the charges referred to only a few pipes of wine. Just as foolishly, within this most democratic of American cities, he reduced the witnesses against him to "poor ignorant people."[28]

In the same month, Benjamin Rush also decided to enter the newspaper battle more directly. He was reluctant to engage a man of such "unworthy character" and did not say much that was new, but he delivered it with his characteristic flair. The profiteering Shippen so easily dismissed was denounced by "the virtue of the army, the declamation of patriots, and the rage of mobs." And Rush claimed that while as many as a thousand died from neglect, Shippen "lived in a constant round of pleasure and dissipation, regardless of the cries and distresses of the sick committed to his care." Rush voiced almost as much disgust for the Congress that had decided to reappoint Shippen head of the medical service; unless they reversed their decision, "we must be an undone people." But Rush aimed his sharpest arrows at Shippen. The manner in which he had abused his sacred responsibilities and "plundered" his country had left him "the butt of the camp, the jest of the taverns, and the contempt of the coffee house."[29]

Rush was not the only local physician to take part in this exchange in the Philadelphia newspaper. James Hutchinson, who would serve as Philadelphia's port physician during the 1793 epidemic, testified that the entire medical service suffered from "want of system." He complained that Shippen failed to provide promised assistance when the sick and wounded were transferred from Valley Forge. And perhaps more damaging, he said that while the director general was a frequent visitor to camp, he never set foot in the hospital, much less made rounds.[30]

But on the other side, Rush's rhetoric forced Philadelphia physician Thomas Bond Jr. to join in. Rush had called out Bond for testifying on Shippen's behalf, despite, according to Rush, frequently complaining privately of Shippen's maladministration. Rush tried to soften the criticism by praising Bond's own character and conduct within the medical service. But Bond would have none of it. Rush's reckless allegations proved him "capable of LYING IN THE WORST SENSE of that opprobrious word" and prove him an "unprincipled man."[31]

Bond's entry into the mix demonstrated just how convoluted and damaging this paper war had become. Bond's father, Thomas Bond Sr., was one of the founders of the hospital and sat on the Board of Trustees of the University of Pennsylvania that had approved Morgan's proposals for a medical school. In 1764, Bond Jr. had married John Morgan's sister Ann; Bond and his wife owned a home alongside Morgan's on Second Street. But now, between Rush's comments and Morgan's allegations that Shippen hid out at Bond's "county seat" while preparing his defense and altering his books, Bond found himself on the other side in his brother-in-law's quarrel.[32]

The Philadelphians following all this in the *Packet* could not have missed how nasty it all had become—the city's medical elite hurling charges at one another with accusations of fraud and profiteering, malpractice and neglect. Shippen clearly got the worst of it. But Morgan did not come off all that impressively either. He may have felt that he traveled the high road, but there was more than a hint of resentment in his attacks on the man who had replaced him; his campaign in the press was far too transparent in its determination to avenge the wrong he believed done him by Shippen. And even though Morgan's case might have gained steam as he presented his evidence month after month, his increasingly strident tone betrayed the smallness of his motivations, the vindictiveness behind his crusade.

In December, after four months of this nonsense, Francis Hopkinson had had enough and submitted a biting satirical piece to the *Packet*. Writing under the penname of Calamus, he complained that in recent months, the paper had lost its sense of purpose. No longer a "vehicle of intelligence," it had surrendered its pages to "private contempt and calumny, to the great abuse of the liberty of the press and dishonor of the city." So that the paper might return to its "original design," this lawyer and future federal judge proposed that a new court be established. Rather than air their small-minded grievances in the press, neighbors could try all cases of "affronts, slights, abuse, scandal, sander, calumny" before a special magistrate. It would be a simple process, he wrote. The grievant need only fill out a declaration stating that "my friend and fellow citizen . . . is a rogue, a rascal, a villain, a thief and scoundrel; that he is a murderer, a robber, a plunderer, a highwayman, a footpad and a cheat; that he has committed sacrilege, blasphemy, forgery, fornication, adultery, rape, sodomy and bestiality; that he is a tory, a traitor, a conspirator, a rebel and a rioter . . . a speculator and depreciator . . . a mean, dirty, stinking, sniveling, sneaking, pimping, pocket-picketing, d——d son of a bitch." And, of course, all this was to be "construed in the most opprobrious sense of the words."[33]

How many others shared Hopkinson's irritation is not known. But at least one person, John Dunlap, owner and editor of the *Packet*, seems to have gotten the message. Within weeks of this piece's appearance in the *Packet*, William Shippen resigned. Morgan immediately prepared a celebratory essay. "I have been able to serve my country effectively in driving from his fast-hold in office, an unprincipled and corrupt servant to the public," he crowed. But the *Packet* would apparently have none of it. This final piece in Morgan's campaign did not appear in the newspaper; instead, the vindicated doctor had to publish it personally as a broadside.[34]

In the years following the war, Morgan, Shippen, and Rush reestablished their positions at the top of Philadelphia's medical community. By 1783 all three had been named to the medical school faculty at the newly chartered University of the State of Pennsylvania.[35] They made rounds in the hospital and maintained private practices. But the tensions between Shippen and Morgan and Shippen and Rush festered. A more firmly established medical community might have weathered all this—dismissed it as the idiosyncrasies of its highly talented leaders. But this bitter acrimony at the top was only part of the story. Among the rank and file, less sensational but more pervasive tensions rippled through the profession. A series of larger structural changes within the practice and consumption of medicine dealt more fundamental challenges to the authority and coherence of the medical community.

It is important to remember that medicine as a profession was still struggling to establish itself in America at the end of the Revolution. Philadelphia's medical school, founded in 1765, still produced only a handful of physicians—far more entered practice through the traditional process of apprenticeship. And unregulated by any sort of licensing or examination process, this traditional path to practice opened the door to incompetence and fraud. Moreover, the fluid conditions of colonial society created an opportunity for any aspiring young immigrant to define himself and his credentials. In America, an ambitious young man with a month's training in a London apothecary shop could call himself a physician; a ship's barber could declare himself a surgeon.[36]

At an even more fundamental level, medicine was changing during these years. The eighteenth century saw the emergence of medicine as "a consumer item or commodity" in both Britain and America as "the business sector of medicine" expanded and deployed "new sales techniques and aggressive advertising." To a certain extent, this commodification of medicine offered opportunities for physicians willing to adapt, but it also filled the medical marketplace with people and products that weakened the status of physicians and undermined the monopoly over medical care they hoped to establish.[37]

One opportunity granted physicians during these years was smallpox inoculation. For centuries, some form of "variolation" had been practiced in Africa and Asia. Infectious matter taken from the active pustules of a victim was inserted into small incisions, usually on the arm, or dried and inhaled through the nose. The inoculee would generally suffer through a mild case of smallpox but was subsequently immune from reinfection for life. The practice gained currency in Europe in the early eighteenth century, and grew widespread after Robert Sutton refined the procedure during the 1760s. Sutton "discovered" that by extracting the infectious material from another inoculee, rather than a natural victim, patients developed an even more mild case and the survival rates of inoculation rose to 98 percent.[38]

Sutton tried to keep a lid on his methods—he and his sons would get wealthy inoculating tens of thousands. But in 1767 Thomas Dimsdale, an English doctor, animated by a sense of "duty," published a tract that spread the Suttonian method through Europe and across the Atlantic. Inoculation was not without its critics. Some argued that it violated the providential order; it was not for humans to interfere with the secondary causes through which God did God's work. But more commonly, critics complained that inoculation actually placed communities at greater risk for disease. Throughout the process, the inoculees were contagious but still well enough, at least during the incubation period, to go about their regular routines. Abigail Adams took advantage of Boston's temporary lifting of its prohibition of the procedure during the summer of 1776 to inoculate her children and herself—but this did not prevent her attending a public reading of the Declaration of Independence and later boasting that she did not miss a single church service while she waited for the infectious material to do its work.[39]

Moreover, those most at risk were the poor. Inoculation was not cheap. During the 1760s prices ranged from two to five pounds for the service; to inoculate his family of five a middling tradesman would have to spend roughly 50 percent of his annual income. As a result, the opposition to inoculation often contained a populist edge—while more affluent folks gained protection from disease, the middling and poor were actually placed at greater risk. Understandably, opposition to inoculation became violent more than once. In 1721 opponents firebombed Cotton Mather's home after he pressed Boston physicians to inoculate for smallpox, and in 1774 residents of Marblehead stormed and destroyed the inoculation hospital set up at Cat Island.[40]

Defenders of law and order criticized the "mob" setting fire to the Marblehead hospital, and later critics have suggested they were "anti" inoculation, in some sense anti-science. But their motives seem to have been more complex. Their real complaint was with the privately funded, limited distribution of the lifesaving lymph. After town leaders concluded that a plan for general inoculation, which was widely supported, was too costly, private groups established the hospital on Cat Island, which was prohibitively expensive. Moreover, the safeguards put in place to prevent recent inoculees from mingling with the unprotected population were poorly enforced, leading to a smallpox outbreak in the town. As Samuel Adams later argued, Marblehead's citizens resorted to violence "deliberately, and I may add rationally" only after the "men in power had rendered the destruction of that property the only means of securing the property of ALL."[41]

In other words, far from expressing resistance to the new medical options, the events at Marblehead demonstrate how far common people would go to secure some degree of control over the medical landscape—and the breadth of opportunities available to a physician who could find ways to meet this demand. For the first time in history, the medical community had developed an effective response to an epidemic disease, staking out an unprecedented role for themselves in the area of preventive therapy. And more than just enhance their reputations, inoculation offered physicians significant financial rewards. These were especially great in a city like Philadelphia where physicians could inoculate without restrictions. This was not the case in other regions. Inoculation was prohibited in Charleston, South Carolina, and severely restricted in Virginia. New York City and most New England cities and villages banned the procedure as well. As a result, Philadelphia physicians enjoyed a steady stream of out-of-colony customers anxious to be inoculated against the century's greatest killer. The opportunities were especially welcome for young doctors trying to build a practice. John Morgan and Benjamin Rush both developed healthy inoculation practices early in their careers. But they were not alone. Inoculation may have generated as much as 20 percent of

Philadelphia physicians' annual fees. During the spring, the income from these services might have approached 50 percent of all incoming fees.[42]

The benefits for doctors, however, were double-edged. Patients gained more than just protection from disease—they discovered a new form of autonomy as consumers. While the basic procedure was fairly standard, physicians surrounded inoculation itself with varying regimens. Many forced their patients through cleansing diets and mercury purges before actually introducing the infectious material. Pricing could vary as well. Some physicians offered group discounts; Rush experimented with complicated contractual arrangements. And as a result, patients enjoyed a new, somewhat unprecedented autonomy as consumers of medical services—they played a more active part in their medical choices and made informed choices from among a range of competing options.[43]

In this regard, inoculation was part of a growing list of medical services and products available to consumers in British North America. Patent medicines, in particular, allowed consumers the chance to select from dozens of premixed medicines and raw drugs to self-treat their various ailments.

Until the seventeenth century, Europe's medicine chest was largely unchanged—physicians drew on many of same herb-based remedies used for centuries. But after 1600 exploration in Asia and the New World led to the introduction of hundreds of new remedies, and some, like ipecacuanha and Jesuit, or Peruvian, bark were actually effective in treating ailments ranging from digestive disorders to malaria. These new drugs contributed to the rising status of apothecaries, but many of these drugs, premixed and bottled, were delivered directly to the public. By the mid-eighteenth century hundreds of patent medicines crowded the shelves of grocers and booksellers—and as they did medical treatment became "synonymous with taking drugs." Europe's growing corps of medical practitioners was not able to stem this drug-taking tide. It was hardly in apothecaries' interest to do so, and as physicians' own conventional therapies were far from foolproof, they could not convince the public to abandon the new products. As a result, physicians entered into what has been labeled a "collusive relationship" with the new medical products. They prescribed and promoted the new medicines themselves, transferring some of their own rising authority to the new therapies, and in the process gave medical self-care a tremendous boost.[44]

Britain's North American colonies were not untouched by all these developments. Light in weight, easy to transport, the profit-promising new drugs and patent medicines quickly found their way to America. Daffy's Elixir Salutis was advertised in the *Boston News-Letter* as early as 1708, and by the Revolution some seventy-five patented medical items had been advertised in American papers. Philadelphia played a prominent role in this multitiered trade; most large merchants and physicians relied on large companies for their supplies, but many small traders—British, German, and Dutch—sent their small lots via consignment in the trunks of passengers. These small lots quietly made their way past customs and onto the shelves of small shopkeepers.[45]

People seeking to self-diagnose and treat were also provided with new literary tools. During the eighteenth century several new medical manuals were written and published for the layperson. Some of these, like John Wesley's *Primitive Physick*, adopted tones and medical positions contrary to the established medical profession, but most others, like William Buchan's *Domestic Medicine*, were written by physicians and toed a fairly conventional line. Buchan, for example, believed that providing laypeople with detailed descriptions of diseases, as well as advice on causes and prevention, would advance conventional therapeutics while reducing superstition and quackery.[46]

The availability of these literary and pharmaceutical tools for medical self-management changed the health care landscape. Self-medication may have provided a first line of health defense for centuries, but in the eighteenth century the new tools gave self-treatment a more commercial as well as a more authoritative character. Self-diagnosis was now confirmed by leather-bound manuals, and self-medication was facilitated by a vast assortment of premixed cocktails in brand-specific bottles. Imported from Europe and promoted within advertisements that stressed their creator's "professional" credentials—Dr. Buchan's Domestic Medicine, Dr. Sanxay's Medicine, Dr. Paschall's Golden Drops—the new products made medical self-management not only more convenient but also more "scientific."

The newspaper ads hawking these patent medicines, elixirs, and raw drugs tell an important part of this story. Readers of Philadelphia's papers were invited to buy Baron von Swieten's Worm Destroying Sugar Plums, Dr. Sanxay's Medicines, Turlington's Balsam of Life, Harper's Female Pills, Dr. Hill's American Balsam, Dr. Ryan's Sugar Plums, Dr. James's Fever Powder, Keysers Pills, Bateman Drops, Maredant's Drops, Walker's Jesuit Drops, and Peruvian bark. For those interested in compounding their own drugs, jalap, calomel, gum opium, quicksilver, distilled vinegar, salt petre, and camphor were regularly listed among the stores of "fresh capital drugs" available for purchase.[47]

The sheer volume of drug advertising suggests that this was a highly lucrative market—and most physicians tried to cash in. As part of a 1765 package of reforms, John Morgan proposed that physicians leave the drug mixing to apothecaries and elevate their own status by restricting their practices to consulting and prescribing. But while his colleagues might have agreed that compounding drugs was a lesser skill, they also knew that the drugs they sold represented a significant part of their incomes. Refusing to surrender the lucrative drug business to all the others crowding the field, physicians were nonetheless not quite willing to compete in the newspapers with these "lesser" vendors for customers. And although they sat on the sidelines, the medical marketplace—and the nature of the competition physicians faced—evolved around them.[48]

In the decade before the Revolution physicians faced their biggest competition in the drug market from apothecaries and merchants. A handful of apothecaries advertised frequently in the press; an almost equal number of merchants regularly announced the arrival of fresh shipments of patent medicines and drugs. But as virtually all of the patent medicines were imported from England, the coming of war in 1775 brought this trade to a halt. A few enterprising merchants, like Nicholas Brooks and bookseller John Sparhawk, managed to stock a short list of patent medicines and pills. But these sorts of ads were rare. Clearly a market for medical products remained. And some unconventional providers tried to step into the void. An itinerant physician named Dr. Yardell offered treatments at his medical warehouse for wens and cancers—and anticipating the medical needs of men at war, aggressively promoted his "antivenereal essence." Recently widowed Elizabeth Weed advertised her services—she had been putting up medicines for the late Dr. Weed for some time—and would continue to fill prescriptions for the public. It is not clear whether these individuals managed to prosper with the coming of peace, but they did signal that the medical market was in transition and that consumers were ready to turn to new providers for their medical supplies.[49]

With the restoration of peace, British patent medicines and drugs returned to America. By the fall of 1783 a half-dozen merchants were announcing recent arrivals of fresh drugs and patent medicines. Rose and Pickens, Tarrasson Brothers and Company, Daniel Tyson, W. Poyntell, and Isaac Bartram all hawked everything from Dr. Hill's American Balsam to opium. But largely missing from the list of advertisers were the apothecaries that regularly advertised before the war. Whereas they had accounted for roughly half of all drug advertising before 1775, they were outnumbered in the postwar press better than five to one. In fact, by 1785 advertising suggests that the market was all but dominated by merchants—Jackson and Smith, Sharp and William Delany; Donnaldson and Coxe; William, Morris, and Stanwick.

A few apothecaries did eventually assume a more aggressive marketing posture. But by 1793 the most prominent newspaper presence was a new category of pharmaceutical merchants: "druggists" and "chemists." It is not entirely clear if this shift represented a narrowing of commercial interests or a strategic relabeling. William Delany, who had distributed a variety of drugs and medical instruments for years, now introduced his wares before the public as "William Delany, chemist and druggist." Merchants Jackson and Smith, who included a large collection of fresh medicines and medicine chests in their wares in 1785, presented themselves in 1793 as "druggists and apothecaries." Isaac Bartram, who had included a line of drugs and medicines within an assortment of dry goods in 1785 under the simple banner "Isaac Bartram," in 1793 listed his goods under the new label "Isaac Bartram and Sons, Chemists and Druggists." While some of these identified themselves as apothecaries as well, more significant is the number who advertised themselves simply as druggists—and addressed themselves directly to the retail market. Betton and Harrison, "wholesale and retail chemists and druggists"; William Delany, "chymist and druggist"; John White, "druggist and chemist"; and Goldthwaite and Baldwin, "druggist and chemist," all made their products directly available to consumers.

These "druggists," or wholesalers-turned-retailers, who offered chemical solutions to people's medical problems, were not unique to America. Britain's medical marketplace reflected the same structural shift. But in both countries this shift demonstrated more than a relabeling of providers. Unlike physicians who dispensed drugs after completing a formal education or apprenticeship, and unlike apothecaries who also served apprenticeships before compounding the public's drugs, druggists served no apprenticeship and pursued no trade-specific education. Just as disturbing for their better-trained medical competitors, druggists sold their drugs at lower prices. In response, British apothecaries launched a campaign against untrained "quacks" and formed the General Pharmaceutical Association in 1794 as a vehicle, in large part, to attain some statutory restrictions on druggists and their practices.[50]

The reaction of American apothecaries and physicians was far less coherent. But they recognized the threat to their tenuous place in the community. For druggists stole more than market share; with their aggressive advertising and extravagant promises they encroached on the authority and professional turf of the physician. They offered free advice, lower prices, and a willingness to sell their wares independent of any sort of physician's prescription. "Chymists" and druggists like Townsend Speakman were willing to put up doctors' prescriptions for their customers, but they were just as willing to bypass the physician altogether and compound "family receipts."[51]

It was an increasingly complicated problem for physicians. The proliferation of patent medicines and self-treatment manuals dramatically increased consumers' opportunities for self-care. The elaboration of a more extensive medical marketplace filled with druggists and chemists willing to operate independent of the conventional medical establishment and undercut its practitioners in their pricing placed the incomes and status of physicians at further risk. There was no chance for any sort of monopoly over health care—and the sort of tidy pyramid envisioned by Morgan thirty years earlier, with regular physicians presiding over a credentialed community that included apothecaries and surgeons, seemed increasingly out of reach. Instead, consumers, with new tools, new information, and willing suppliers, seemed positioned to turn the physician-patient relationship entirely on its head.[52]

Benjamin Rush summed up the dilemma faced by physicians in a 1789 address on "the duties of physicians." Speaking to his students at the conclusion of the term, he advised them to live on farms. The humble lifestyle would ingratiate them with their patients—and provide them with a second source of income. Acknowledging that the commercial demands of the medical marketplace placed physicians in awkward positions vis-à-vis their patients, he suggested that farming would enable them "to practice with more dignity" and protect them from "the trouble of performing unnecessary services to your patients." Perhaps most importantly, the independence provided by a second source of income would "change the nature of the obligation between you." Within this new medical marketplace, the power had shifted to the consumer. Loaded with options, able to purchase medical products and advice from a variety of sources, consumers had gained the upper hand. They knew "they are the channels of your daily bread." But if an alternative source of income could be established, the power dynamics might turn, and patients would once again feel "the obligation is on their [the physicians'] side for health and life."[53]

From a physician's point of view, it was good advice—and perhaps some of Rush's students took it. But eighteen years later Rush's concerns about the transfer of power within the medical marketplace had only increased. He now lectured his students explicitly on how to cultivate business honorably, and more tellingly he included a lecture on the "duties of patients to their physicians." Patients should have just one physician—that is, all members of the family should see the same physician and that physician should be consulted for all cases, major and minor—they should not shop around, they should not change physicians without substantial cause, they should not seek the counsel of a second physician without the explicit approval of their first. And if another physician offered his services, patients should spurn the offer, rejecting even the "friendly visits" of an outside physician. In other words, a physician's monopoly over a household's medical care should be complete, extending to even the psychic health of the patient. "Debt, love, guilt, intemperance, domestic troubles"—these all bore upon a person's health. Nothing should be hidden from the physician. More importantly, nothing should be confided to another source.[54]

Rush's objectives were obvious. Physicians needed to establish their monopoly over medical care in the community. And since it was doubtful many patients were actually listening, it is clear Rush's real audience was the young doctors in attendance. They needed to set these standards, demand this from their patients, and also demand this from one another. They needed to respect each others' turf—not poach patients, not accept competing consultations. That Rush was delivering this talk two decades after the first suggests that the power dynamics had not changed, and that consumers still governed the medical marketplace. That he was still lecturing medical students—preaching to the professional choir—suggests that physicians were still not doing their part to teach their patients the ground rules—respecting one another's turf—so that patients would behave themselves.

Rush may have been surprised that physicians were not acting in a more collegial fashion: still poaching clients, accepting consultations, undercutting colleagues through competitive pricing structures. But in retrospect it is clear that the institutions were simply too weak. And even if Rush could make his students toe the line, too many of the city's physicians lay outside the college's influence. Although Philadelphia could claim a better-educated medical corps than other American cities, the majority of the city's physicians did not possess a medical degree. Despite the growing number taking courses at the College of Philadelphia (soon to become the University of Pennsylvania) Medical School, the particular structure of the school precluded the establishment of any real monopoly over medical practice.

In adapting the Edinburgh model of medical education that John Morgan brought to Philadelphia, American educators soon recognized the need to make some concessions to American conditions. Therefore, Edinburgh's three-year course of study was reduced to two and its six-month semester to four. Yet even with these changes, only a minority of the city's physicians took the time to attend, and as late as 1810 fewer than 40 percent of those attending actually completed the full course of study and took the M.D. Perhaps most critically, the school failed to secure any licensing authority during these years; aspiring physicians remained free to pursue their training via apprenticeship. And despite the school's efforts to win support for strict nomenclature for various types of health care providers, practitioners routinely self-labeled themselves and their practices. Physicians trained at the College of Philadelphia or Edinburgh posted the same shingle and embraced the same title—physician—as apprenticeship-trained and even self-taught practitioners.[55]

John Morgan had tried to address the lax professional standards and porous professional barriers in 1766 by proposing a companion institution to the medical school. He recommended that a medical society, modeled after Britain's Royal College of Physicians, be chartered to examine and license candidates to the profession and oversee professional conduct. But he ran into considerable opposition from local practitioners. And as the debate evolved between Britain and its colonies over the next decade, with its rhetoric about mercantile barriers to trade, the creation of an institutional monopoly over practice grew even more untenable.[56]

In the years following the Revolution, as threats from apothecaries and druggists increased and as internal divisions within the profession multiplied, a group of physicians decided it was time to revisit the concept. They founded Philadelphia's College of Physicians. It was, however, just a shadow of the institution originally envisioned—and a pale imitation of the British inspiration. Most significantly, it made no attempt to win powers to examine and license aspiring physicians. Instead, despite its referential name, it aimed primarily to function as a medical society. It would collect and publish papers and speak for the medical community on matters of public concern. The college did aim to increase "uniformity and order" within the profession—but given the absence of any control over access to the profession this ambition is telling. Unable to monitor who entered the profession, the college hoped to at least improve the behavior and relations of those within it. After several decades of professional acrimony, bitter feuds among its leading figures, and growing tensions resulting from competition and client poaching, the college hoped to impose some internal code of ethical practice. It is not insignificant that the most extensive section of the college's bylaws were the "regulations to promote order"—more specifically, the rules governing the treatment of another physician's patients.[57]

Founded in 1787—just six years before the yellow fever epidemic presented the college with its greatest opportunity and challenge—in the short term the college did very little. After much pressure, members begrudgingly donated volumes for a library. It issued a couple of collective statements on public health—one on intemperance, a second in opposition to the dangerous "general illumination" planned for George Washington's presidential inauguration. In 1789, at the request of the Pennsylvania legislature, the college issued some general advice on contagious diseases, recommending that incoming vessels secure certificates of health before being allowed to dock in the city's harbors. And in the summer of 1793, the college issued its first collection of papers; it would not issue another until 1842.[58]

Perhaps the most portentous episode in the College of Physicians' early history occurred in 1788 when it heard an ethics charge brought against Dr. John Foulke by Dr. William Currie. Foulke had been called in to treat one of Currie's patients while Currie was out of town. Upon his return, the patient chose to remain under the care of Foulke. Currie accused Foulke in effect of poaching his patient and violating the ethical code of the college of which they were both members. In the end, the college suggested the entire episode resulted from misunderstanding and took no action—except recommending that all future ethics cases be handled in private. Established largely to mend professional fences and, in the process, advance the profession's reputation, the last thing the doctors needed to do was air their laundry in public.[59]

If they had only learned.

4

The Fractured Response to the 1793 Epidemic

DIVIDED AT THE TOP—AND threatened from below, it is not surprising that Philadelphia's medical establishment responded badly to the epidemic in 1793. Their institutions filled with conflict, their attempts at reform ineffective, and their monopoly on medical authority undermined by new pharmaceutical providers and empowered consumers, no wonder they squandered the opportunity presented by the medical crisis. Rather than responding with a single voice, they bickered; rather than putting aside their differences long enough to forge an authoritative response that might have calmed the community and advanced their prestige, they engaged in a public slugfest that shattered their credibility and undermined public confidence in the profession.

It is telling that the facade of professional unity disintegrated almost immediately once the crisis began. When Mayor Matthew Clarkson summoned the College of Physicians to his office on 25 August, they must have recognized the golden opportunity handed them to strengthen their corporate authority. Further, they must have realized that a united, confident, and authoritative response would do much to advance their profession's status. But amazingly, they equivocated. With the public anxious, with many laypeople already recognizing the signs of yellow fever, the medical elite divided in their diagnosis of the ailment plaguing the city and refused to label it by name, calling it only a "malignant and contagious fever." And unable to reach agreement as to cause or cure, they offered only the sort of general advice suitable to most any medical challenge. They called for the establishment of a "large and airy" hospital and urged citizens to stay out of the sun and evening air. They suggested that people dress "appropriate to the weather" and avoid intemperance, and that the doors of the sick be marked and the streets kept clean.[1]

Benjamin Rush actually wrote the report that was adopted and published in the papers on 27 August. And given that he had concluded a week earlier that yellow fever was in town and that it stemmed from the rotting coffee dumped on Ball's Wharf in July, the report's lack of specifics is somewhat surprising. Yet perhaps (and somewhat out of character), he wrote the more vague report in hopes of preserving consensus within the college and thus its authority. If so, the strategy backfired, for since the medical establishment refused to speak with clarity, others filled the newspapers over the next week with their homespun analyses.

Some, like "Veritatis," focused their efforts on diagnosing the disease: it was nothing more than "a modification" of the influenza that was troubling the city, they insisted. More were ready to recommend the cure. "A. Hint" suggested that it was a simple matter of collecting the garbage more frequently. "A Friend" recommended that the streets be doused with vinegar. One writer to the *Federal Gazette* urged residents to spread a thick layer of fresh dirt on their floors to absorb the infectious toxin; another argued that it could be blasted from the air by firing cannons at regular intervals. Pharmacists offered a host of vinegar-based elixirs. And one writer to the *Daily Advertiser* took the vinegar cure a step further: they recommended a daily washing of the temples and loins with a mixture of vinegar, wormwood, rue, and lavender. For good measure, individuals should snort some of the concoction up their noses.[2]

The most useful advice in the papers came from "A.B.," who suggested killing all of the mosquito larvae hatching in rain tubs. The author did not suspect any connection between mosquitoes and yellow fever but felt they were a nuisance, "distressing to the sick and troublesome to those who are well." Yet no doubt this advice was lost amid the cacophony. And in fact, Rush's elation on discovering his cure was tied, in part, to his interest in replacing this untutored noise with a scientifically based "medical principle." Once convinced that his cure was effective, he shared his discovery with everyone who would listen. Yet not every Philadelphia physician embraced his purge-and-bleed recommendation—and within days of Rush's discovery, the dissent went public.[3]

The first physician to challenge Rush was William Currie. His short pamphlet, first advertised in the *Gazette* on 7 September, did not flatly deny Rush's theory on the origins of the fever; in fact, he conceded that filthy, putrefying matter could generate contagious toxin. He was just more suspicious of the muck lying beneath Water Street homes than the coffee sitting on the nearby dock. But he more aggressively challenged Rush on the reach and treatment of the disease. Whatever its origins, the miasma did not represent a floating toxin capable of infecting people at great distances; instead, Currie wrote, its range was limited. Planting a more painful barb, he suggested that Rush's warning of a generally circulating and deadly miasma was contradicted by "the learned of every age and country." Instead, laying the foundation for what would be the "contagionist" position in opposition to Rush, Currie argued that the fever was a "specific contagion" that could only be communicated through direct contact with the sick or by "receiving the breath or the scent of the several excretions of the sick" within the confined air of a sick room.[4]

Given the limited range of the toxin, Currie recommended several preventative steps. To purify the air within sick rooms he suggested the odd combination of good ventilation, house plants, and a constantly burning fire laced with potassium nitrate. And while he conceded that the fever's early stages were inflammatory, and thus might suggest the need for bleeding, the debilitating stages that followed advised against harsh treatment. Instead, he recommended only a mild emetic, like chamomile tea, and various sudorifics that would leach the toxin from the body through sweating.

A few days later, Adam Kuhn piggybacked on Currie's analysis. The fever was not due to some systemic overstimulation, he argued; it was, in fact, the opposite: a direct, debilitating fever that weakened the system and thus called for gentle treatment. Rather than purging and bleeding, patients should be given chamomile tea and bark (quinine). Purges and laxatives of any kind, even those more gentle than the mercury prescribed by Rush, should be avoided. Adding a postscript to this challenge,

Secretary of the Treasury Alexander Hamilton submitted an endorsement of Kuhn, who, Hamilton claimed, had successfully treated him and his family during their bout with yellow fever.[5]

Rush wasted no time in responding. He immediately published in the *Federal Gazette* a description of his cure, accented by some critical comments on the therapies recommended by Kuhn and his associate Edward Stevens. Rush had consulted with the latter, he told readers, because Stevens had some experience with fever in the West Indies, but using Stevens's methods, three-fourths of his patients had died. Clearly, Philadelphia's yellow fever was different than the Caribbean variety, and therefore Kuhn's and Stevens's experiences were irrelevant. Rush followed up the next day with a more elaborate defense of his analysis, and since he was too busy to see all those requesting his services, he published directions for self-administering his purges. He reassured residents that there was no need to flee the city as the disease was "under the power of medicine." And he published a public letter to the College of Physicians admonishing the body for its "contrariety of opinion" and warning that "intrepidity in the use of the lancet is . . . as unnecessary as it is in the use of mercury and jalap."[6]

But Rush's critics were not cowed. Kuhn submitted his own letter on 13 September, suggesting that Rush's warnings of a citywide epidemic were unfounded. Of the sixty patients Kuhn had treated for fever, he wrote, only seven had yellow fever, while the rest suffered from more common remittent and intermittent fevers. And Currie echoed Kuhn's suggestion that the yellow fever was far less widespread than Rush suggested: "Have we all got the yellow fever in our bodies, only waiting for some exciting cause to put it into action? . . . By no means. The disease which Dr. Rush calls the yellow fever . . . is only the fall fever."[7]

Daily, the debate between the doctors grew more intense and personal. Rush suggested that Kuhn read Thomas Sydenham. The "English Hippocrates" had firmly established that two fevers of "unequal force cannot coexist long"; while a "monarchical" or "despotic" fever like the yellow fever was in town, all others were quickly driven out or absorbed by the ruling contagion. Rush also cited the results achieved by other doctors using his treatment—Dr. John Pennington reported curing forty-eight of forty-eight patients using Rush's cure while losing all six patients Pennington had earlier treated with Kuhn's wine and bark. The evidence was overwhelming, Rush concluded. Therefore, Kuhn should keep his fatally flawed opinions to himself rather than "adding to the mortality of the disorder."[8]

Throughout September and October, the *Federal Gazette* was filled with arguments between the two medical camps. Rush and his allies posted their success rates (Dr. John Porter claimed thirty-seven cures in three days); Kuhn's supporters, like "A Physician," offered elaborate evaluations of Rush's methods before labeling them dangerous. Far from scholarly and respectful, both sides all but accused the other of murder. Rush's recommendation of purging and bleeding promised "certain death," wrote Currie. Doctors choosing to bleed their patients might just as well slit their throats, wrote another Kuhn supporter. Kuhn's and Currie's advice, answered Rush, would only succeed in "desolating three-fourths of our city."[9]

Rush ultimately claimed a victory of sorts. He boasted that his mercury purge proved increasingly popular as the epidemic persisted. And judging by the number of apothecaries carrying his powders, he may have been correct. But clearly, the real loser in the contest was the medical profession. Handed the opportunity to strengthen its authority and advance its corporate identity, Philadelphia's College of Physicians failed miserably to construct a coherent and convincing response.

One illustration of this failure was the persistence of lay commentary in the *Federal Gazette* through the crisis. Not forced from its pages by a unified authoritative voice, lay analysts received equal space within the public arena and retained, quite possibly, equal credibility among the general public. Alongside Rush's explanation of inflammatory fevers and Kuhn's analysis of debilitating agents, "X" described their own instantaneous infestation with the disease: "It pressed suddenly through my whole frame . . . excited a blowing like a horse that has been overrode." And uninhibited by medical "authorities," they described their own self-treatment with liberal doses of molasses that quickly produced "great and frequent discharges from the bowels . . . always accompanied with great discharges of wind." Suggesting that common sense and shared experience might prove more trustworthy than "trained" professionals, they noted "it is a known fact" that molasses "has not its equal for removing wind from the stomach and bowels."[10]

"Y" more directly entered the debate between physicians. Was it not possible that Rush's treatments might actually spread the disease even while curing it, they asked. After taking Rush's powders, victims "sit with ease in the Temple of Cloacina, voiding what they suppose to be the disease in embryo; and at the same time inhaling the noxious effluvia from the black stools and discharges of vomit (from some one of his diseased family) which just before were launched from the chamber pot of the nurse."[11]

But perhaps the most significant comment came from "A Citizen," who summed up the community's confusion and growing disgust with the medical profession: "From such a contrariety of sentiments, what are we to conclude, or how shall we act? . . . This is no time, sir, for party disputes. . . . There have been sufficient time for experiment and from the results thereof to fix . . . which method has been most generally beneficial."[12]

The disappearance of the fever—not any sort of professional discipline—brought the worst of this squabbling to a close. But the larger debate persisted. Over the next several years several Philadelphia physicians published major works on yellow fever and the 1793 epidemic, as well as those that quickly followed. These works illustrate the divisions that persisted on the origins of the disease and the most effective treatment. But they also reveal that even within these broad camps considerable differences existed. While lines were drawn, they were not yet hard and fast; Philadelphia's medical community was more fragmented than rigidly polarized. Ideas about disease were still protean. And just as important, they reveal that Philadelphia's physicians were not content to turn passively to inherited ideas. Ultimately, they may not have been able to move beyond central beliefs about "corrupted air" that had dominated Western medicine for centuries. But in their compilation of disease histories and their nuanced conclusions about the fever that had ravaged their city, they demonstrated a commitment to adding a new level of precision to their scientific inheritance.

For example, Jean Deveze, the physician hired to oversee the hospital at Bush Hill, staked out a position that was in many ways similar to Rush's. He argued that the fever was inflammatory in the early stages and targeted, most dangerously, the brain. For these reasons, bleeding was useful when quickly applied. Deveze also insisted that the yellow fever originated locally and was not imported—and he was emphatic that it was not contagious. Like Rush, he explained that the body was sensitive to external impressions, most powerfully the air, which he labeled a fluid. When "corrupted" or "charged with miasmata," the body's intricate operations were placed at risk. This was all standard Rush, but Deveze added a different emphasis in arguing that some people were more vulnerable than others—those weaker physically or morally—explaining the selective spread of the disease. And this, he argued was the source of the confusion. Since the disease was not universal in its impact, many assumed it was not universal in its reach—and thus spread only by contact. But this was not the case. The source of the disease, an atmosphere corrupted by miasma, had indeed spread over the city, but the stronger constitutions of many protected them from its influence. As proof, he offered the examples of many doctors, nurses, and caregivers who spent hours in the sickrooms breathing the supposedly contagious air of victims and yet never acquired the disease themselves. Their survival offered proof that yellow fever was not contagious, "only epidemical."[13]

Deveze clearly supported the most essential parts of Rush's analysis. But he was not in lockstep with Rush. While Deveze bled patients in the first inflammatory stage of the illness, he took fewer ounces. And he shied away from harsh purgatives, like calomel and jalap. In general, his treatment plan aimed to assist patients through its dangerously inflammatory initial stages and then assist nature in its efforts to bring about recovery. He was not unwilling to act, to produce the "salutary crisis" when nature, "overcome by the force of the disease, remains without action." But there was a time to take a backseat to nature. Deciding when to act and when to do nothing was "the physician's art."[14]

David de Isaac Cohen Nassy, Philadelphia's first Jewish physician, shared the essentials of Rush's diagnosis but carved out a distinctive emphasis. He traced the disease to a local miasma fed by the carcasses of dead animals and insects and stewed in the city's peculiar summer weather. The stink rising from local burial grounds also played a part. Ignoring an emerging semantic distinction between contagionists and miasmacists, he suggested that all epidemics, regardless of origins, were contagious. Like Rush Nassy also recommended that patients be bled in the early inflammatory stages—but never more than twice. And he joined Deveze in discouraging the use of mercury purges. Dissections conducted at Bush Hill had revealed "the havoc those violent medicines . . . had caused in the stomach and intestines."[15]

Nassy's most distinctive contribution to the discussion was his argument on the diseases' greater impact on local residents. Others had noted the same, but he fit this observation within a Rush-like analysis of disease. Just as the body was responsive to the stimuli that surrounded it, individuals were most sensitive to changes within the atmosphere to which their bodies had grown accustomed. Individuals' "organical constitution has great homogeneity with the air" of their native land, Nassy argued. And thus, they were more susceptible to "the impressions of the putrid miasmas, with which the air is impregnated," unbalancing "that equilibrium of the solids and liquids so necessary to maintain good health."[16]

Felix Pascalis-Ouvière, a French-trained physician who fled Saint-Domingue to Philadelphia in 1793, also published an account of the 1797 epidemic that largely supported Rush's analysis but offered a longer list of the sources of putrefaction—graveyards, wooden wharves, and ancient privies—that converged with the distinctive weather of the previous year to produce the fever. He challenged contagionists by asking why the disease had not penetrated the American countryside, despite the legions of refugees who fled the infected city. And then he further muddied the whole debate by offering his own definition of contagion. It implied nothing more, he argued, than "the transmission of certain principles of disorder, whether conveyed through the medium of the air or by an immediate contact." Perhaps trying to carve out a reconciling position, he suggested that while the disease originated in the city's filth, infected individuals became human incubators: "in them the contagious miasmata regenerate and multiply" and "acquire more malignancy when they are propagated by the channel of diseased human bodies."[17]

On the other side of the debate, William Currie further established himself as the most vocal "contagionist" and leader of Rush's opposition—a fact that galled Currie's former teacher. He had studied under Rush at the University of Pennsylvania and absorbed the central premises of Rush's theories. The dissertation on autumnal remitting fever Currie published in 1789, which he dedicated to Rush, regurgitated Rush's Brown-based views that "the whole phenomena of life may be reduced to one simple cause, the stimulant operation of certain powers, applied to a certain property of living bodies . . . the excitability of the animal system." Disease, Currie parroted, is based on the "excess or defect of excitement" leading to too much "vigor" or "debility."[18]

Yet by 1793, Currie was no longer the fawning student. He had been the first to trace the disease not to a ubiquitous miasma but rather to a "specific contagion." And he was among the most industrious in constructing a natural history of the epidemic that traced the disease to specific ships carrying cargoes and emigres from the island of Saint-Domingue, plagued with yellow fever and insurrection. Currie was far from alone in these conclusions. James Hardie followed Currie's lead in labeling Rush's rotting coffee theory "chimerical" while asserting there was "no doubt" that the fever was introduced by the passengers and crews of the *Sans Culotte, Flora,* and *Amelia.*[19]

These men were on the right track. Colin Chisholm, a British military physician, writing in 1795, may have come even closer to the truth in identifying the ship *Hankey* as the primary source of the deadly infection. The ship had left England in April 1792, carrying a group of well-intentioned but terribly naive settlers to the island of Bolama, off the west coast of Africa. Inspired by, in the words of Chisholm, a "fanatic enthusiasm for the abolition of the slave trade," their goal was to build a colony using free African labor to demonstrate the potential for more humane alternatives to slavery. But the expedition ran into problems almost immediately, including alienating the neighboring Canabac community on which they would depend. By fall, most of the settlers had succumbed to one illness or another, and in November the few survivors decided to return to Britain on the *Hankey*, carrying several active cases of yellow fever and hordes of disease-carrying mosquitoes.[20]

But they had to take an indirect route home. With French privateers attacking British ships along the African coast, the refugees were advised to sail to the West Indies, where they could join a larger fleet traveling to England. They stopped first at Barbados—with yellow fever breaking out within days of their arrival—then island hopped across the Caribbean. The *Hankey* reached Saint-Domingue in June with the Haitian Revolution raging all around them. And with white planters looking for passage off the island, and the *Hankey*'s captain, John Cox, more than willing to take on fee-paying passengers to cover expenses, the ship set sail, laden with a new batch of nonimmune arms and legions of hungry mosquitoes, reaching Philadelphia in July.[21]

While Currie, Harding, and Chisholm were right in recognizing that the disease came to Philadelphia on ships from the West Indies, they were just as blind as Rush to the role of the mosquito in the transmission of the disease. In fact, one of the ships they blamed—the *Amelia*—brought to Philadelphia not just refugees but also the cargo of rotting coffee that Rush identified as the source of the disease. In a sense, then, while differing on the infectious agent they carried—coffee or refugees—they were equally blind to the vector actually responsible for its transmission.

Still, Currie in particular has provided historians with an attractive counterpoint to Rush. He may have missed the role played by the mosquito, and he may have been wrong in believing that the disease was being spread by person-to-person contact. But within his identification of a "specific contagion," many have found the seeds of a more modern understanding of disease, the hint, perhaps, even of a germ theory.[22]

The earliest scholarly account of the epidemic contributed to this characterization of Currie by suggesting that the two physicians "were at opposite poles." But the truth is more ambiguous. Currie's understanding was inchoate, at best, far from modern and far closer to Rush than the intensity of their argument suggested. While Currie's repeated emphasis on "specific contagions" and his tracing of certain diseases to "morbid *matter*" suggest to some that he recognized diseases as distinctive conditions produced by discrete infectious entities, his larger body of writing reveals that his ideas were more cluttered and rooted in their own time. While some diseases might be "permanent and constantly existing," he argued that others, including most putrid fevers, were "generated and propagated." The greatest danger was the "febrile miasmata" rising from the shores of stale ponds and marshes; those most at risk were the poor living in crowded conditions and breathing "vitiated air."[23]

In other words, Currie's more general understanding of disease was quite similar to Rush's. And even one of Currie's most significant points of departure—his conviction that the disease was imported from the West Indies—may have been inspired less by scientific precociousness than by the position he staked out just a year earlier in what he most certainly believed was his greatest contribution to medical thought. In *An Historical Account of the Climate and Diseases of the United States,* Currie reviewed the climatic conditions of each region and the diseases these conditions produced. He devoted the largest section to Philadelphia—and for local readers, the conclusions were gratifying. The Delaware River was kept fresh through tidal motion; most of the surrounding lowlands had been drained and were under cultivation. The city's streets were kept dry and clean, and dirty water was carried off by underground aqueducts and sewers. In other words, the environmental sources most commonly responsible for putrid fevers and other ailments were not present in Philadelphia.[24]

The city was not immune to illness, conceded Currie. Yet his review of the most common ailments reveals that he subscribed, in large part, to an eclectic set of ideas typical of the period. The wealthy were afflicted by several conditions rooted in the "joint effects of intemperance and indolence"; the poor suffered a range of fevers bred by their squalid living conditions. Women's health was compromised by too little meat, too much tea, and too frequent clothing changes, which led to constant changes in body temperature. Everyone exercised too little and, consequently, deprived their solids of the motion needed for proper circulation of the fluids. But—and here he staked out a more distinctive claim—the "principal" cause of disease in the state was the "sudden vicissitudes of weather."

Abrupt shifts in the temperature from extraordinary heat to bitter cold, as many as six times within a twenty-four-hour period, left the body vulnerable to illness.[25]

Six years later Currie made the same argument in explaining the cause of cholera. Warm summer weather caused "a deficiency of vigour in the several functions of the human body, and especially in the functions of the liver." The body was thrown into even greater imbalance when the weather abruptly changed—and consequently a simple action, like eating too many "crude vegetables," produced a morbid reaction that led to too much bile being secreted into the alimentary canal causing cholera.[26]

The point is not that Currie was not a disciplined thinker—it is that even those who seemed to be tending toward more modern or sophisticated understandings of disease were often just as archaic in their thinking. And their notion of "contagion" did not bear any real similarity to those that would emerge three-quarters of a century later.

The closest thing to an exception might be Isaac Cathrall. Born in Philadelphia but medically trained in London and Edinburgh, Cathrall was another prominent contagionist—in fact, he and Currie coauthored an analysis of a later yellow fever epidemic in Philadelphia and Wilmington, Delaware, that reflected their common belief that the disease was an imported contagion. Like Currie, Cathrall's contagionist argument emphasized the limited range of the toxic emissions emanating from a sick person. It could only be spread through direct contact with the sick or their belongings, such as woolens, bedclothes, or furs. And when airborne, the toxic emissions of the sick were very quickly "diffused, corrected and modified" by pure air. The contagion he identified was oddly discriminatory. Foreigners, the deranged, and "idiots" were largely immune to its effects. Yet more clearly than Currie, Cathrall tiptoed toward a more modern understanding of disease. He suggested that the "*matter of contagion*" was in some sense organic, or more specifically "quiescent," until activated by heat and other things.[27]

In the years following the epidemic, Cathrall conducted research aimed at identifying the actual agent of contagion. The "black vomit" spewed by victims at advanced stages of the disease was a likely candidate, so Cathrall conducted extensive experiments on the coffee-ground-like stuff. After pursuing a series of experiments designed to determine the chemical nature of the substance, he fed vomit-infused beef to cats and dogs, and bread soaked in the gunk to chickens. None experienced any ill effects. The cats exhibited a stronger "propensity to combat . . . a malicious spirit" but nothing more morbid. The chickens, Cathrall reported, actually developed a preference for the vomit-laced feed. Cathrall also conducted human tests. He dipped his hands in the vomit and applied it to his lips and tongue. To make sure that the tests were conclusive, he applied vomit from several different victims. He also convinced a friend to submit to the same tests. The conclusion, for Cathrall, was definitive. His extensive testing demonstrated the "inactivity" of this substance. It was no more than "an attendant" to the real causes of death—direct or indirect debility—and not the carrier of the contagion.[28]

Four years later Stubbins Ffirth published the results of the experiments he had pursued in Cathrall's wake. Similarly intrigued by the role that black vomit might play in the transmission of yellow fever, he, like Cathrall, fed the stuff to dogs and cats before actually injecting it directly into the jugular vein of a dog. After that he pursued similar experiments on himself, swabbing portions of the discharge into open cuts on his arms. He also heated the vomit, inhaling its vapors, before ingesting the dehydrated residue.[29]

Ffirth emerged convinced, like Cathrall, that the vomit played no part in the transmission of the disease. Neither adventuresome investigator succeeded in identifying the actual agent of infection, the organic material that actually transferred the disease from one person to another. But their efforts to do so offer a tantalizing glimpse of the sort of research that might have moved Philadelphia's physicians toward a more useful understanding of the disease, a hint of the possibilities had curious physicians like Deveze, Nassy, and Pascalis-Ouvière subjected their deductive analyses to a similar form of laboratory research, and a hint of the possibilities had the city's physicians more generally managed to substitute collegial investigation for partisan invective. And the idiosyncrasies within the views of all these thinkers reveal the inchoate state of disease theory more generally. While the 1793 epidemic had exacerbated tensions within the city's medical community, medical ideas were still fluid. Orthodoxy had not been established; even among fellow travelers, there were disagreements.

While medical professionals wrestled to understand the disease that plagued them, the more general public discourse—the commentary in the press from both professionals and laypeople—over yellow fever evolved as well. The disease became a regular visitor to the city over the next five years but except for a brief time in 1797, the public controversy was muted. That does not mean Philadelphia's physicians had buried the hatchet or reached some sort of consensus. When the fever returned in late summer of 1794, the old divisions were still evident. Rush sent a letter to the Philadelphia Committee of Health warning that yellow fever was back in town and that his purge-and-bleed therapy continued to be effective. And, as he complained in a letter to John Redman Coxe, Kuhn and his supporters, most notably Caspar Wistar and William Currie— or "the Kuneans"—continued to oppose him. Yet neither camp launched a concerted public campaign. Instead, the newspapers—and public attention—focused on the threat to Philadelphia posed by the yellow fever epidemics in other cities.[30]

New Haven, Connecticut's health crisis was the first to alarm Philadelphians. Word of a spreading fever and rising death count reached Philadelphia on 20 August. And by 1 September Philadelphians had been alerted to an even more severe epidemic in Baltimore. Pennsylvania governor Thomas Mifflin quickly ordered the inspection of all ships that had passed within thirty miles of New Haven. New York's Committee of Health similarly suspended all intercourse with the infected town. And no doubt alarmed by the speedy isolation of the Connecticut town, Baltimore officials tried to downplay the severity of its health crisis before it found itself similarly isolated. Despite this, Philadelphia residents seized on every hint and rumor of an epidemic that reached their ears—and by mid-October all trade and travel to the Maryland city had been suspended.[31]

There is no evidence that the public reaction was engineered by Philadelphia officials anxious to steer public attention away from the health problems in their own town, but the preoccupation with health crises outside the city did seem to absorb most of the public anxiety. While Rush's warnings of a local threat drew little public response, the attitude toward Baltimore voiced within public meetings and letters to the press was loud and uncompromising. Calls for a more tempered response to Baltimore's crisis—more evidence of the severity of the epidemic—were summarily dismissed. And Baltimore's pleas for moderation were met with charges of a coverup. The Maryland city should take a lesson from Philadelphia, one Philadelphian argued: during the 1793 epidemic "there was no attempt made for concealing its ravages."[32]

Philadelphians responded in similar fashion the following year when the disease broke out in New York. The New York Committee of Health tried to contain the rumors of yellow fever when the disease appeared in mid-August 1795—the reports were mere "old women stories." But by the end of month, officials had to concede that some sort of fever was present, even though, they insisted, it was confined to just one small district in the city and there was "no decided evidence of a specific contagion, or of a nature peculiarly infectious." The New York Medical Society, similarly recognizing that continued trade with Philadelphia hinged on whether the disease was contagious, claimed it was communicable only within "the sphere of its original and local atmosphere."[33]

For Philadelphians, the question of contagion also became paramount. As yellow fever morphed from a local to an external threat, the debate evolved as well. Questions regarding origins persisted but only to the extent that they affected questions surrounding dissemination. How might the disease be spread? Could it be transported? In other words, what had been hotly debated in the past, when the disease was actually among them, was replaced in the newspapers with a less contentious consensus. That yellow fever was contagious, wrote Governor Mifflin in suspending trade with New York, was "no longer a matter of doubt." Philadelphia's Board of Health put the matter more bluntly: "It is of small moment to the point in question, whether the disorder was imported or originated in the city from local causes, it is sufficient to prove it contagious."[34]

But while this new consensus served to unite Philadelphians as they crafted a response to Baltimore and New York, the détente between the city's warring medical factions did not last long. In the summer of 1797, following yet another yellow fever outbreak, two newspapers—William Cobbett's *Porcupine's Gazette* and John Fenno Jr.'s *Gazette of the United States*—came after Rush, his theory of the disease, and his purge-and-bleed therapy with a vengeance.

Both papers launched their first salvos on 18 September. In Cobbett's, "A Tavern Keeper" mocked Philadelphia's "Dr. Sangrado," who had reduced the complexity of modern medicine to "the very simple system of copious bloodletting and comfortable evacuation." Fenno's *Gazette* printed a letter from "A Citizen," who complained that Rush's belief that yellow fever was generated locally, rather than imported, had done more damage to the city than the disease itself—and added that the theory was born in the "bewildered imagination of some whimsical man."[35]

Over the next two weeks the two papers presented letters, supposedly written by readers, and editorial comments mocking Rush and his theories. Cobbett poked relentlessly at Rush's "medical puffing"—the manner in which he and his followers promoted one another through letters in the press—and lamented that "the times are ominous indeed, when quack to quack cries purge and bleed." When some of Rush's supporters like Dr. James Tilton of Wilmington, Delaware, rallied to his defense, Cobbett turned his venom against them. Tilton was nothing more than "the trumpet, the underling, the mere barber-surgeon of the Master Bleeder." And revealing that politics, probably more than science, informed Cobbett's crusade, he called Tilton an "incorrigible democrat." Meanwhile, Fenno's *Gazette* piled on. In its pages "Paracelsus" argued that bleeding and purging—this "lunatic system"—had "destroyed more than the sword." Another contributor suggested that "if the reign of blood is to continue, we shall soon see our butchers and farriers aspiring to seats in the College of Physicians."[36]

Incensed by the attacks, Rush brought a libel suit against the two papers on 1 October. But if he thought merely filing the suit would silence the papers, he was wrong. An editorial in the *Gazette of the United States* now argued that "Dr. Sangrado" was threatening the constitutional rights as well as the lives of Philadelphians. But while the papers were not silenced, the character of the attack did change as local physicians and citizens reentered the controversy, revisiting for the first time in years the questions first debated in 1793.[37]

William Currie took the lead in defending the contagionist position that yellow fever was spread only through direct contact with a victim or breathing their exhalations. Even more dangerous were the residues deposited in bedding and clothing. These "fomites" were actually more lethal in their power and the cause of the disease's easy transport.[38]

Currie also went undercover with a letter he signed as "a member of the College of Physicians" that took more viciously personal aim at Rush. Learned men recognized that Rush's ideas were "insane." His idea that the entire atmosphere was loaded with the toxin was the product of "a whimsical brain." And as the crisis and Rush's sense of importance grew, Currie said, Rush raced through the streets shouting to those even casually encountered, "You've got it! You've got it!" After a cursory assessment of public health in one city, Currie added, Rush ordered his lieutenants to "bleed and purge all of Kensington." He even enlisted "illiterate Negro men to bleed and purge."[39]

Merchant Benjamin Wynkoop and Dr. John Redman Coxe, Rush's former student, rallied to Rush's defense. The allegations of frenzied, knee-jerk diagnosis were the stuff of mean-spirited gossip. And the two "illiterate Negro men" were Absalom Jones and Richard Allen—two "worthy leaders" within the Black community who had "great success in curing the fever after most of the physicians were confined by it."[40]

Coxe also answered Currie's vicious rhetoric in kind. He ridiculed Currie's complete misreading of the 1793 epidemic's severity in its early weeks; on 12 September Currie had written there were fewer than forty or fifty cases in the entire city, yet records indicate there were eighty-one deaths on that day alone. Noting that Currie had actually embraced portions of Rush's analysis in prior years, Coxe suggested that Currie's brain was "not only whimsical but versatile too." And he argued that Currie's cowardly anonymous attack on his former teacher revealed a convenient neglect of all former obligations. Hadn't Currie studied under Rush and dedicated his dissertation to the man? Hadn't Rush forgiven Currie for the way he turned against Rush in 1793 and ignored how Currie had abandoned his patients by fleeing the city during the 1797 epidemic? Currie's mind, Coxe concluded, had become "a sink into which a number of filthy streams have flowed . . . offensive to everybody but fatal to himself alone."[41]

The vitriol within this exchange during the fall of 1797 was reminiscent of the paper war of 1793. But on deeper examination significant differences emerge. Far fewer people entered this new debate. Currie was the only physician to speak out on behalf of contagionism, and Coxe was the only physician to rally to Rush's defense. More significantly, the new controversy was in many ways more political and personal than medical—Cobbett in particular seemed animated by a vehement dislike of Rush and his politics. Cobbett joked during the controversy that he would like to see "half a dozen democrats stuffed with straw" and put on display at Charles Willson Peale's museum along with the other "curiosities."[42]

And the public that in 1793 had ping-ponged between frustration with the professionals' lack of certainty and serious engagement with the questions in dispute now appeared more interested in the debate as entertainment. Even Cobbett, who insisted that he was animated by his concerns for his readers' health, interested solely in protecting the public from the lunatic system of Dr Sangrado, was willing to sell advertising space in his paper to pharmacists peddling Rush's purging powders. Alongside condemnation of Rush's violent debilitating therapy, Cobbett ran regular ads hawking "Doctor Rush's bilious purging powders and pills . . . the best mode of treating the bilious yellow fever."[43]

In other words, the 1797 controversy suggests that the debate which had engaged the public just a few years earlier had settled into comic parody, fair game for satire and entertainment. This explains why in 1798 the public response to yet another outbreak was muted. In fact, no longer enflamed by the polarizing debate among professionals, the general public embraced a mushy blend of all the etiological and therapeutic ideas circulating within the medical community.

"X" is representative. Noting that professional opinion was still divided on the question of origins, he offered up the wisdom of Solomon in suggesting that since there was danger "from both foreign and domestic matter," steps should be taken to remove both. Suspicious vessels should be quarantined at a safe distance from the city to prevent the importation of infectious material, and streets, sewers, and docks should be cleaned as the noxious vapors arising from rotting animals and vegetative matter were "sources of diseases and death."[44]

"Mentor" followed with a more extensive but similarly hybridized analysis that traced recent epidemics to imported contagion animated by the "particular circumstances" of the local environment. Chief among these circumstances was a corrupted atmosphere infused with the "putrid exhalations from dead animal and vegetable substances."[45]

And while there might have been something intellectually deadening in this resort to mushy hybrids and trend toward rolling elements of previously contested theories into a comfortable amalgam that settled nothing, the laypeople constructing them could hardly be faulted. The medical professionals were still unable to articulate a reassuring consensus—and a few even had simply thrown in the towel. "The best skills of our physicians and all the powers of medicine," conceded Philadelphia's Health Office, "have proved unequal to the contest with the devouring poison."[46]

With the medical community still divided and many physicians showing signs of intellectual exhaustion, demoralized by a public willing to mock their authority and haphazardly cobble together a variety of homespun theories and remedies, the stage was set for some group or institution to provide direction and clarity—a voice that could speak to medical practitioners and laypeople alike. As Philadelphia recovered from yet another yellow fever outbreak, the stage was set for the emergence of a new voice of authority.

5

America's First Medical Journals and the Battle for Authority

WHEN ELIHU HUBBARD SMITH died in 1798 at the age of twenty-seven, his friend Samuel Miller eulogized the young intellectual as "one of the most enlightened and promising that ever adorned the annals of American science." Henry May, the preeminent historian of the American Enlightenment, was as effusive in celebrating the literary circle that surrounded Smith as "perhaps the most brilliant of all the . . . organizations of earnest and enlightened young men" during the early republic. The "Friendly Club" did indeed include a number of important literary figures—Noah Webster, William Dunlap, Charles Brocken Brown. Yet Smith was their undisputed leader, and from a distance, the praise heaped on him is hard to figure. He made some small contributions to an early but not distinguished journal, the *Echo*. He published some insignificant poetry as well as collected and edited an anthology of American poetry that would be forgotten had it not been simply the first.[1]

Smith realized his greatest contribution to American intellectual life as the founder and editor of the *Medical Repository*. Yet in this there is a certain irony. He himself was a poorly trained physician and lethargic practitioner. Moreover, the *Repository*, while it remained the nation's most influential and important medical journal for several decades, was under Smith's watch a poor model for other professional journals. The first volumes were narrowly partisan, focused on canonizing Benjamin Rush's theories of disease in general, and yellow fever in particular. Issue after issue defended Rush's theory of local origination and promoted his

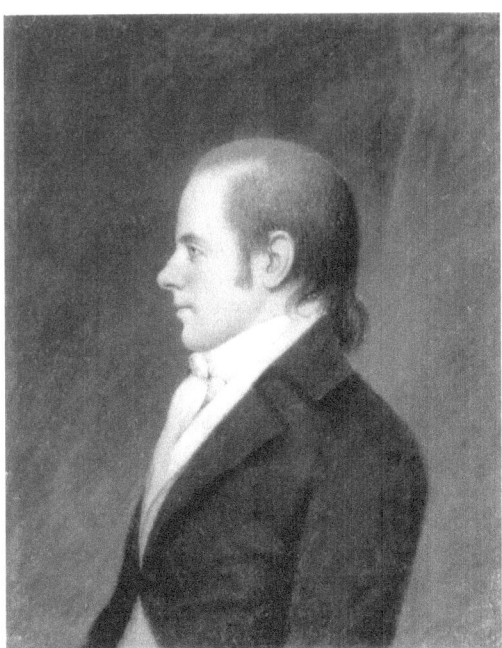

Elihu Hubbard Smith, founder of America's first medical journal, the *Medical Repository*, by James Sharples, ca. 1797. (Litchfield Historical Society, Litchfield, Connecticut)

therapeutic regimen of purging and bleeding. Smith himself wrote many of these articles—like Rush he asserted that properly diagnosed and quickly treated, yellow fever could be reduced to a minor threat. But in September 1798 Smith contracted yellow fever as it spread through New York, and on 19 September he died.[2]

There's no denying that Smith was something of a prodigy. He entered Yale at the age of eleven and took his degree in 1786 when he was fifteen. While in New Haven he joined one of the college literary clubs and participated in a series of dramatic productions and forensic exercises. A biographer has suggested that his relative youth—the average age of his classmates was seventeen—prevented his participating in the whoring and gaming common to eighteenth-century college life. Nor did he participate in the student "rebellion" that followed President Ezra Stiles's attempts to increase the rigor of the school's year-end exams. Smith did join in the more general rebellion within the student body against orthodox

Christianity. But for the most part, he completed his Yale years in unspectacular fashion, distinguished mainly by his being at the time the youngest person to take a Yale degree in the school's history.[3]

But the precociousness that had led to Smith's early matriculation now presented something of a dilemma. Too young at only fifteen to enter a profession, his father debated his son's prospects before deciding to complete his education by reversing the normal progression and sending him to preparatory school. Smith spent the next year at Timothy Dwight's school at Greenfield Hill where, by Smith's account, he grew more intellectually and morally than he had during his four years at Yale.

Believing himself better educated—and, if nothing else, a year older—Smith returned to his home in Litchfield where he studied under a local doctor. At the same time, he apprenticed in his father's apothecary shop. But in 1790 Smith decided to add some formal training to his medical toolkit by enrolling in the College of Philadelphia. He registered in Benjamin Rush's course in the fall, but this course, which ended in February 1791, was probably the extent of Smith's formal academic medical training. There is no record of his taking any other courses, nor did he take a degree or write a thesis. Instead, at the end of the term, he turned his attentions to his dream of becoming a writer.

Three months later Smith was on the move again—first back home to Litchfield, and then to Wethersfield, Connecticut. He half-heartedly tried to establish a medical practice but failed, and dabbled in the local theater and played around again with being a writer, contributing to the *Echo*.

In 1793 Smith returned to New York City, again with a two-pronged ambition. He joined the practice of a local doctor and began editing an anthology of American poetry. While there was greater focus to his professional and literary efforts this time around, neither proved all that impressive. The doctor with whom Smith partnered actually turned over the entire practice to the younger doctor, but in short order it had withered to just a few patients. And the anthology Smith put together is now viewed as insignificant. He did invest some energy in the local manumission society and became a member of the city dispensary—but amid all this, his most important decision may have been to keep a diary.

Launching the project in 1795, Smith brought to the task a healthy ego. "My attainments," he wrote, "certainly surpass those of most persons of my age." And after a somewhat lackluster start, he promised that his third volume, commenced in September 1795, would provide an even more vivid "picture of my mind . . . fraught with richer treasures of reflection, more enlarged narrations of events, & more copious transcripts of scenery & fiction." But for all the ambition, his journal proved a largely unsatisfying list of project proposals and daily events, ultimately disappointing even to himself. In increasingly frequent entries he lamented his "habits of indolence and gossiping," his "universal torpor" resulting from too many friends and too many distractions.[4]

By late 1795 Smith had decided that he was a failure and his prospects were thin: "My intellect seems ponderous & my body nerveless. I am unfit for any noble purpose." In his more hopeful moments Smith planned the narrative, the grand tale that his indolence would ultimately serve—a history of his mind "from error to truth, from despair and inactivity to assurance & energy." And finally in the summer of 1796 he hit on the idea that would allow him to complete this narrative and earn him a place in the history of early American letters: he proposed the creation of a journal, to be called the *Medical Repository*, dedicated primarily to the study of the epidemic and endemic diseases of the United States.[5]

A couple of factors had converged to shape this vision. Noah Webster had recently published his collection of letters on yellow fever. Smith had contributed to that anthology several letters he had written to William Buel; it was perhaps Smith's most sustained intellectual effort to date, and he was proud of his contribution.[6] Webster's announcement that he would not publish a second volume left the field open for a similarly aimed sequel. In addition, Smith's recent appointment as a staff physician at New York's general hospital had both clarified his vocational path and deepened his sense of inadequacy. The "consciousness of my own ignorance . . . especially of my professional ignorance" had been "redoubled" by the daily demands of his patients.[7]

The journal he proposed thus provided an opportunity to increase his professional knowledge while satisfying his own need for a larger purpose—a project well suited to the young doctor better at thinking than doing, better at talking about medicine than actually practicing it.

In late July Smith prepared a circular letter describing his proposal. In it he promised that the journal would be intellectually unbiased, a literary space for the presentation of all theories and points of view. But Smith himself was becoming even further entrenched in a Rush-based assessment of disease in general and yellow fever in particular. In Smith's contribution to Webster's collection, he had argued that there was absolutely no proof of importation; in fact, the attempt to find a foreign source was a "ridiculous vanity." Instead, the "efficient cause, the causa sine qua non . . . would be clearly discerned as depending on local circumstances." And upon receiving Rush's fourth volume on yellow fever, Smith sent his former teacher praise and supportive evidence drawn from his New York experience. The cause of yellow fever was undoubtedly local, he insisted, concentrated in seaports not because it was imported but because these low-lying areas were ideal breeding grounds for the putrefaction-spawned miasma that caused the disease. The most effective treatment for the fever was liberal purging and bleeding; one of his colleagues, Smith added, had to good effect taken 176 ounces of blood from a patient over a two-week period—as much as a quart at a time.[8]

Thus, while Smith might have pledged to give all positions a fair hearing, he was also committed to vindicating his former teacher and establishing his ideas as medical orthodoxy. He was incredulous, he told Rush, that skeptics remained: "You will yet live to taste the sweet reward of all your painful sacrifice . . . by leading the way to the use of this remedy." In fact, this became the "great work" he now set before himself—"to labor towards the general diffusion of correct ideas, or subjects the most important to national health."[9]

Within days of writing this, Smith began what would be his first major article for the journal he envisioned—an analysis of the plague of Athens. When it appeared in the first issue of the *Medical Repository* in August 1797, Smith's examination of the ancient plague was a historically based defense of Rush's disease theory. Athens's plague was locally generated and despotic; it drove out all other lesser diseases. And just as "local causes" triggered this ancient pestilence, "local causes may generate a yellow fever in Philadelphia and New York."[10]

Smith's article was not the only commentary on yellow fever in the inaugural issue. Rush's recently published account of Philadelphia's 1794 epidemic was favorably reviewed. In fact, the editor commented that the evidence of local origins had "long since removed every doubt on this question." And a Dr. Morton's study of the fever's history in England demonstrated that foreign disease studies were unnecessary, as there was plenty of evidence of "the materials of mischief growing up and acquiring malignity under our own eyes." The second issue of the *Medical Repository* continued the defense; it led off with a letter from Dr George Davidson explaining that yellow fever only arises where water stagnates and putrefaction occurs. The greatest danger, he warned, followed rain, which broke the crust of stagnating ponds, allowing the "noxious vapour to escape."[11]

In its first year, the *Repository* permitted a few dissenting voices—but only so as to dismiss them. Alexander Hosack's criticism of purging and bleeding was unequivocally denounced by the editors. Some communications from Philadelphia's College of Physicians, which continued to oppose Rush and his theories, were reprinted, but they were set against a much longer letter from Rush and his supporters and another glowing review of a Rush treatise. The effectiveness of Rush's therapeutic regimen was settled, the editors declared to those who might still be missing the point; his opponents' arguments were "inconclusive and fallacious."[12]

Smith died in 1798 but the *Repository*'s apologetic mission continued. In May 1799 Samuel Brown added a chemical analysis of the impact of putrefaction in his account of Boston's recent epidemic. Stagnant water, rotting meat, and clammy winds robbed the air of azote (nitrogen), "the cause of all malignant or pestilential diseases." Henry Channing considered the culpability of marshy lands and overflowing privies before concluding that a pile of rotting fish caused New London's yellow fever outbreak. The stink was "like none previously experienced." And Joseph Browne suggested that modern chemistry might offer a solution to the ancient miasmatic theories—planting more trees in the vicinity of effluvia-generating filth would restore the proper chemical balance to vitiated air. The new editors, Samuel Mitchell and Edward Miller, made similar gestures toward balance. They included an announcement of William Currie's latest memoir of the recent epidemics but quickly noted that despite all the overwhelming evidence, Currie stubbornly clung to debunked theories that the disease was imported.[13]

Over the next several years, the narrow defense of Rush's disease theory only grew more rigid, and on the pages of the *Repository* uncontested. After ten years the journal remained unashamedly partisan; in fact, by 1807 the apologetic form had crystalized—the local reports that buttressed Rush's theories followed a predictable template. A Dr. L. Wheaton's account of a yellow fever outbreak in Providence began with a review of the region's geography and flora. Particular attention was paid to the "seat of the yellow fever"—the wharves and waterside communities in the western part of town. The outbreaks that had occurred in 1797, 1800, and 1805 had been most severe there, not because these areas received incoming vessels but because of the "unwholesome exhalations" emanating from these low areas. Like many other accounts of the period, Wheaton's also rebutted, ship by ship, the theories of importation—investigating and then clearing the vessels that had been blamed by contagionists for importing the disease.[14]

Like earlier editions, international voices were occasionally added to the apology. J. M. Beguerie stated that "malignant distempers" were "native productions." And he explained that confusion arose as merchant ships often generated disease-breeding conditions due to "cargo perishing and putrefying beneath the decks." But while disease might arrive by ship, its cause was the same sort of putrefaction that could be produced in swamps, marshes, privies, or cellars. Importation theories were nothing more than an expression of "national vanity," a jingoistic attempt to blame foreign sources for local conditions.[15]

The decade-long crusade of the *Medical Repository* is undeniable—determined to establish etiological orthodoxy, its voice was rigidly partisan and uncompromising. There were other medical journals launched during the period; the *Repository*'s control over the professional literary turf was not uncontested. But the contributions of these others to the professional discourse on disease were less significant, either because they were too eclectic, too short-lived, or in their greater commitment to more balance and greater breadth, less insistent.

The *Philadelphia Medical and Physical Journal* was launched in 1804 by Benjamin Smith Barton. Before suspending publication in 1809, the journal proved more balanced in its review of the controversies surrounding yellow fever. William Currie, as an author absent from the *Medical Repository*, submitted a large report for the first issue of the Philadelphia journal. Still the most determined and vocal contagionist, he tried to convince readers that mercury and bleeding were all but abandoned in Philadelphia's city hospital and called for the strengthening of quarantine laws by citing the findings of the latest College of Physicians report.[16] At the other end of the spectrum, George Shattuck of Boston offered to the pages of the journal a John Brown–type analysis of the human body that implicitly affirmed Rush's theories. The body, Shattuck said, was a "physical machine operated upon by physical agents, the force of whose action depends upon the excitability of the subject."[17]

Somewhere in the middle, Dr. Thomas Smith of Loudon County, Virginia, endorsed much of Rush's analysis of the disease and its origins but concluded that venesection was a risky, and often counterproductive, form of treatment. And Dr. Tudor Harris of South Carolina, reporting on the outbreaks occurring in Charleston since 1793, suggested that putrefaction had to be coupled to some "insensible qualities of the atmosphere" to produce an epidemic. Yellow fever was undeniably of local origins. But this not unprecedented riff on Rush's theories emphasized the "peculiar unknown modification of the atmosphere, evidently the consequence of the heats of summer," as an essential ingredient to the mix producing disease.[18]

The short-lived *Medical and Agricultural Register* (1806–7), published in Boston, was also less doctrinaire than Smith's *Repository*—but it was also less sophisticated. Articles on disease and treatment were printed alongside advice on pruning trees and curing butter. An essay insisting on the effectiveness of cold-water therapy for treating fevers ran next to an article on removing bots from horses. Yet in its pages one can still see how the growing orthodoxy was filtering down. One lay contributor commented on the dangerous effects of noxious vapors from wells, cellars, and fermenting liquors. Another observed that the "effluvia of dirty cottages and dirty rooms, are of like nature with pestilential vapours."[19] Yet while the *Register*'s readers seemed to be settling in with Rush's miasma-based theory of disease, their views varied on the efficacy of bleeding. Dr. James Mann reported that liberal bleeding and purging had proven successful in treating croup. But Drs. L. Danielson and E. Mann concluded that purging regimens, including calomel, had been ineffective in treating the disease which attacked Medfield, Massachusetts. And their experimentation with bleeding proved disastrous. Even though they took only one ounce from the jugular of a fifteen-month infant, "the effect was unfortunate."[20]

In fact, the other journals appearing during these years, like the *Philadelphia Medical Museum,* launched in 1805 by Rush's student John Redman Coxe, may be as useful in tracking popular attitudes as professional ones. In addition to revealing the steady, even if challenged, dissemination of Rush's ideas, they reveal that medical professionals were engaged in a constant debate over diagnosis and therapy with their patients. Ironically, while the *Repository* joined other medical professionals working to establish medical orthodoxy, their patients worked to assert their place in the diagnostic and therapeutic conversation.

Within the case studies submitted by physicians to the *Philadelphia Medical Museum,* they complained frequently that their patients resisted their counsel and often flat out rejected the treatments they prescribed. A mother refused all courses of treatment for her child that might induce nausea. A woman so incapacitated by dropsy that she could barely walk rejected "all internal remedies and even bleeding." The parents of a young girl suffering from convulsions refused to let her doctor perform the "division of the scalp" he advised, allowing only the application of blisters. A father insisted that his son receive the "vegetable remedy" (Geranium Maculatum) he had learned from an Indian, rather than the surgery his physician recommended, when the boy severely cut himself with a hatchet. One of a Dr. McDowell's patients refused several treatments prescribed for his pulmonary consumption as they left a foul, even painful taste in his mouth. The patient was buttressed in his position, complained

McDowell, by the "officious interference of some benevolent old ladies, who lay claim to a large portion of experience."[21]

While patients like these seemed to feel that their doctors were prescribing too much, others complained that their physicians were not doing enough. Reverend Samuel Smith summoned a doctor to address the coughing fits that seized him while preaching, fits so extreme that he coughed up blood. The physician administered a light bleeding. But when this did not produce the desired effect, Smith asked that he be bled again—and more vigorously. The doctor refused, believing it excessive. But Smith pressed him, as he "would rather die bleeding from the arm than from the mouth." Reluctantly, the doctor acquiesced, but apparently to separate himself from further responsibility, he left his lancet with Smith so he could bleed himself in the future. And bleed himself he did. Over the next ten days Smith used the tool four times a day, taking more than two gallons of blood. By removing so much blood, Smith reasoned, he would remove the "impulse of blood from the wounded part . . . [and] give it time to heal."[22]

Reverend Smith was a keen enough observer of his physical condition to recognize that this extreme loss of blood took its toll. He lost weight and muscle tone and he grew pale and could barely speak above a whisper, but when he did recover his confidence in his diagnostic and prescriptive abilities was strengthened. His health was not perfect—he now suffered from chronic constipation—but to combat this he prescribed himself a daily laxative, again against the advice of his physician, who feared permanent damage to Smith's bowels. But Smith was willing to take the risk; overall, he felt his self-treatment had led to better health. And this, he crowed, despite his having "no medical education and . . . no theory to bias my mind."[23]

A timid physician might also explain a General Martin's decision to develop his own treatment for the bladder "stones" that plagued him for fifteen years. Using a steel wire and incredible grit, Martin fished the wire through his urethra and filed down the recurring stones. He could only work for five minutes at a time—or until the pain became unbearable—but in this way he managed to break up the stones, which were then eliminated through urination.[24]

While northern doctors reported countless examples of patient resistance, southern doctors faced a more complicated challenge to their authority and the lucrative niche within the plantation economy. Asserting that the distinctive physiologies of Black people required specialized treatment, they appealed to slaveowners anxious to protect their valuable workforce. But in many instances, slaves preferred their own healers—men and women who weaved together folk traditions carried from Africa with conventional white therapies to address illness. For white southern doctors, this was problematic enough, but to make matters worse, many slaveowners seemed to place as much and sometimes greater trust in these Black healers than they did in white practitioners. Slaveowners transferred certain medical services more readily to Black healers than others. For example, Black midwives were routinely entrusted with the delivery of white as well as Black children. But many slaveowners were willing to entrust virtually all medical care of their slaves to Black practitioners, usually trained in conventional medical procedures like bleeding and purging.[25]

Physicians clearly resented these various forms of patient independence and worked to overcome this resistance to their authority. And if unable to cajole their patients into compliance, they were not above resorting to deception. William Dewees, America's leading expert on obstetrics, explained that one way to help women through a difficult delivery was bleeding. If an expectant mother was slow to dilate—or if she experienced excessive pain—removing as many as sixty-five ounces of blood would relax her cervix and dull her senses. In more extreme cases, women should be bled until they fainted. But, Dewees complained, many patients were afraid of this approach. And some physicians shared their timidity. Elihu Smith might have been one of these: he suggested the use of tobacco as an alternative. If "thrown up the rectum" the patient might relax (even if this did often lead to vomiting). But Dewees remained fully committed to bleeding—and fainting—even if it required some subterfuge. Most patients would agree to a light bleeding, he explained, and if told they must stand, rather than sit, for the procedure, the likelihood of their fainting increased. So long as he "conceal from them our wish to have her become faint," Dewees explained, he could trick her into this very outcome.[26]

It was not the ideal strategy. Physicians were far more interested in winning their patients' confidence and in establishing via successful treatment their authority over all things medical. And as part of that objective, they sought to change the fundamental beliefs about disease and health, that is, they sought to increase confidence not just in their own abilities but in the efficacy of medical intervention. Dr. T. Watkins angrily recounted the failure of a burn victim's parents to apply the turpentine liniment that he had prescribed. Believing their child's condition hopeless, they ignored his recommendations; only his angry entreaties convinced them to resume the treatment that saved the child's life. And Dewees, when he wasn't tricking his patients, chastised them for not following the recommendations that might preserve the lives of infants born prematurely. There was plenty of evidence to indicate that fetuses delivered as early as the sixth month would survive, he argued. It was therefore a parent's "indispensable duty" to act as though there was a "certainty of their living."[27]

Convincing a skeptical public that more and more illness was falling under the dominion of medical science may even explain the medical journals' fascination with physical oddities and abnormalities, especially those surrounding pregnancy and childbirth. One doctor submitted an account of a headless fetus; another described the removal of a fetus from the side of a fourteen-year-old boy. An "Eboe wench" was forced to deliver her child anally as the fetus had attached itself outside her uterus. And several doctors discussed the possibility of superfetation—one doctor reported delivering a healthy child four weeks after his mother gave birth to a slightly older sibling—and concluded they must have been the issue of entirely separate pregnancies.[28]

These accounts can appear sensational—perhaps even a pandering appeal to the lay readers that journal editors hoped would swell their readership. But there is reason to think these accounts were more political than sensational, intended less to exploit curiosity than to assert the unlimited possibilities of science. In his account of two albino children born to the same woman, Dr. John Vaughan explained that studying the "grievously and wonderfully deformed" paved the way for "remedying the incidental evils of our nature."[29]

Increasing confidence in medical science and establishing the authority of the profession were also clearly a secondary objective in the largest medical crusade of the period: smallpox vaccination. With Edward Jenner's successful development of a vaccine drawn from cowpox, most progressive physicians rallied to the treatment and supported massive efforts to vaccinate entire regions, even empires. But Jenner's discovery did not go uncontested. The most systematic challenge came from William Goldson, a surgeon from Portsea Island in England, whose own research suggested that vaccination provided only very temporary immunity. His conclusions were embraced by skeptics in the United States. But medical journals and the vast majority of physicians contributing articles on the topic solidly supported vaccination.[30]

Edward Jenner's demonstration that lymph scraped from the oozing sores of cows suffering from cowpox and inserted into a small incision on the arm would provide immunity to smallpox was the most significant medical breakthrough of the era. Despite the spread of the Suttonian method of inoculation during the second half of the eighteenth century, smallpox claimed an estimated 400,000 European lives annually—and one-third of all blindness was caused by the disease. But once Jenner's treatment was embraced, deaths from this dreaded disease gradually decreased until it was wholly eradicated by the end of the twentieth century.[31]

Jenner's discovery resulted from his embrace of a longstanding piece of folk wisdom. Among the dairy farmers of certain English counties, it had long been believed that exposure to cowpox protected people from smallpox. Dairy maids claimed themselves immune to the disease after touching the infected sores on their cows' teats and suffering a minor reaction. In fact, some farmers deliberately exposed their children to infected cows—encouraged them to handle the cows' sore-covered bags in order to achieve protection. The medical community largely scoffed at what seemed yet another piece of unscientific folklore. But Jenner, a young man when he took up practice in the rural community of Berkeley in Gloucestershire County, England, in 1773, was more willing to accept the common belief. During a smallpox epidemic of 1778, he recorded the histories of those untouched by the disease and concluded that exposure to cowpox had indeed provided immunity.

Jenner wrote up his findings in a paper that he presented to the Royal Society of London, but it was rejected as inadequately supported. Jenner was actually a member of the society, but he had gained entry on the recommendation of his former teacher John Hunter, largely on the basis of a study of the cuckoo bird. Jenner had no reputation in disease study, and he also suffered from less than sterling credentials. He did study under Hunter, the most respected anatomist of the period, and he served a lengthy apprenticeship, a not uncommon path to a career in medicine. But his mentor, a Mr. Ludlow, was a surgeon, not a physician—and surgery was considered a lesser skill. In fact, other than his studies with Hunter, Jenner had no academic training. To members of the society, it was hard to believe that a relatively poorly trained country doctor could produce a medical discovery of such magnitude.

Jenner remained convinced of his beliefs, but his ability to prove them was complicated by the fact that cowpox occurred neither regularly nor universally. The bovine disease only appeared periodically; it would not resurface for close to twenty years. And it seemed to only attack the cows in some English communities. But when it did reappear in 1796, Jenner went about his research in more deliberate fashion. He began by carefully studying the character of true cowpox. Realizing that many who discredited his work could provide examples of individuals who had been exposed to some sort of cow disease but remained vulnerable to smallpox, he carefully sorted true from faux pox and drew careful diagrams illustrating how to differentiate between different skin diseases. He also demonstrated that the matter extracted from the pox only conveyed protection if taken at a certain phase of the disease's development.

Most daringly, Jenner conducted a series of experiments on people. His first subject was eight-year-old James Phipps. Jenner took lymph drawn from the hand of a milkmaid who had been infected by a diseased cow—Blossom—and inserted it into a small cut on Phipps's arm. Within a few days, the child developed a fever and tenderness under his arm, as well as smallpox-like skin eruptions. But within just a few more days, these had disappeared. Jenner then waited a month before subjecting Phipps to the older process of inoculation. He took live material from a smallpox victim and inserted it into the boy's arm. But Phipps experienced no reaction. The live smallpox virus had no visible effect on the boy.

Jenner repeated the experiment with several other subjects with the same results. Convinced that he had proven that cowpox provided immunity to smallpox, he produced a small pamphlet, published it at his own expense, and circulated it widely. Jenner's conclusions were not without error. Most significantly he argued that the immunity gained in this fashion endured a lifetime. He was wrong about this: immunity thus acquired endured closer to ten to twelve years. But for the most part his conclusions about this new preventative treatment—soon labeled "vaccination" to differentiate it from traditional forms of "inoculation"—were rapidly embraced.[32]

Jenner had his critics. Doctors attached to the Suttonian method of inoculation—and financially benefiting from its place in their practices—questioned his findings. But more significant and impressive were the campaigns launched by philanthropic societies and even nations to vaccinate the public. The most ambitious was sponsored by Spain's King Carlos IV. He commissioned a global vaccination expedition in 1803, under the charge of Francisco Javier de Balmis. Balmis set sail for the New World carrying twenty-six orphan boys who would serve as human repositories for the vaccine. The first pair were vaccinated on the day of departure. Ten days into the voyage, lymph from the small eruptions on their skin was inserted into the arms of the next pair of boys. Through this method of serial transmission, live vaccine was delivered to the Spanish holdings on the Canary Islands and then Cuba, before reaching present-day Venezuela, Panama, Colombia, Ecuador, Peru, Chile, and Bolivia. In Mexico, Balmis collected a second set of young boys before sailing for the Philippines and then China. By the time he returned to Spain in 1813, after a ten-year campaign, the expedition vaccinated perhaps as many as 100,000 persons in New Spain alone.[33]

Similar efforts were launched by the British in the Mediterranean in 1801. And the international crusade made its way to the United States in the person of Boston physician Benjamin Waterhouse. In 1800, using lymph secured directly from Jenner, Waterhouse vaccinated his own children. He also conducted his own experiment to demonstrate the efficacy of Jenner's discovery. Gathering nineteen young boys volunteered by their parents on Noddle's Island in Boston Harbor (the Boston Board of Health had insisted the experiment be conducted a safe distance from the city), Waterhouse vaccinated them with cowpox. Three months later, he inserted matter taken from an active smallpox sufferer into incisions on their arms—the traditional method of inoculation—and celebrated (along with their parents) when not one of the boys experienced any reaction.[34]

Waterhouse's experiment convinced doctors and lay people to undergo vaccination. But meeting the growing demand was difficult. For starters, cowpox did not occur in the United States. To maintain a steady supply of live vaccine, he paid Boston parents to vaccinate their children on a schedule. He also joined others in experimenting with ways to transport the needed material across the Atlantic. The most common was to soak short threads in the lymph drained from sores and then seal these within glass bottles. Others dried the lymph and placed it between slides. Thomas Jefferson, an early supporter of Waterhouse's efforts, placed the lymph he used to vaccinate his family and household, including enslaved people, within a glass container that was then placed in another glass container filled with water to keep the lymph cool.[35]

Waterhouse, like Jenner, encountered some resistance from colleagues attached to the traditional form of inoculation. Many American physicians sought to protect their inoculation practices; others were skeptical about the ability of an animal disease to convey human immunity. And these sorts of questions contributed to a more general malaise surrounding vaccination at the turn of the century. The sorts of ambitious public campaigns launched by Spanish and British authorities in the wake of Jenner's discovery were not replicated in the United States.

The failure is especially curious as inoculation campaigns (using the Suttonian method) had been successfully implemented during the Revolution. For years, the Massachusetts state legislature had prohibited inoculation in the belief that inoculees actually spread the disease by refusing to quarantine themselves during the contagious phase of the process.

But in July 1776 the legislature reversed course and called for the opening of inoculation hospitals throughout the state. Terrified by rumors that the British intended to quash the rebellion by spreading the dreaded disease, state officials called for general inoculation with tremendous success. While 304 people caught the disease naturally during the summer, and 29 died, almost 5,000 people were inoculated with only 28 dying. The mortality rate of less than 1 percent proved the value of mass campaigns.[36]

As commander of the Continental Army George Washington initially opposed inoculation, similarly believing that the net effect would be to spread the disease. Even when confronted with smallpox outbreaks in the ranks, he resisted pleas from medical officers because he feared his already weakened army would be vulnerable to British attack during the process. But in February 1777 he overcame these fears and ordered a general inoculation of his troops through the creation of inoculation hospitals throughout the states.

Beyond their success in protecting troops and civilians, these campaigns asserted the role of the government in protecting public health. In fact, they set the precedent that protecting the public health was a "foundational duty of government." But neither state nor municipal authorities jumped at the chance to provide mass vaccination—of the Jenner type—in the years after the Revolution, despite the fact that the method was safer, produced fewer side effects, and left no collateral scarring.

Some historians have blamed the resistance of physicians who wanted to retain control over the entire inoculation/vaccination industry. Rather than transfer the means and, most importantly, the lifesaving lymph to city officials, they took steps to preserve a monopoly over the procedure and the profit. There is plenty of evidence to support this argument. But it also seems true that the yellow fever epidemics of the 1790s left many skeptical about the basic science behind vaccination. The entrenchment of Rush's miasmatic theories, the belief that all disease was tied to rotting organic material, undermined the contagionist premises of Jennerian vaccination. Most proponents of Rush's ideas carved out a different space for a few diseases like smallpox. But among some, a belief in the all-inclusive power of toxic miasmas contributed to their resistance to aggressive vaccination campaigns.

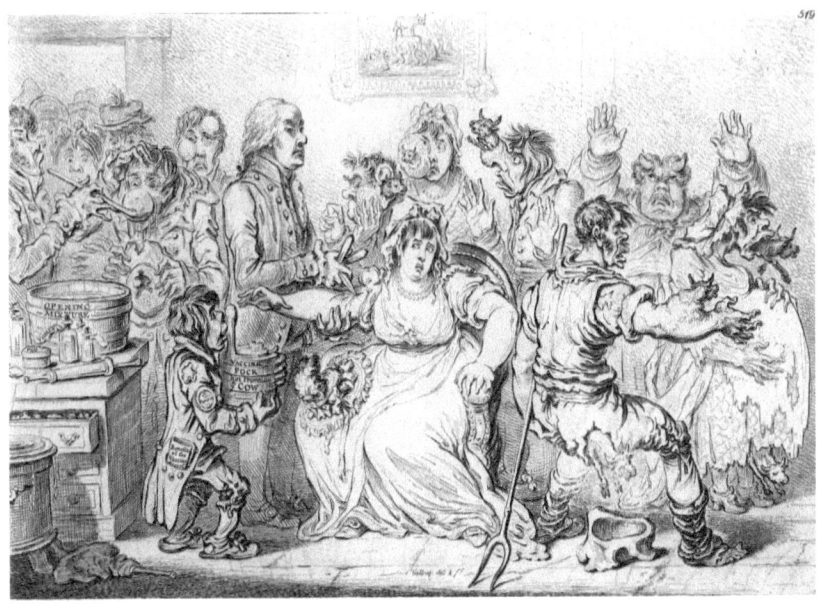

"The Cow-Pock—or—the Wonderful Effects of the New Inoculation!" published by the Anti-Vaccine Society of London, 1802. (National Library of Medicine)

Yet while state and local governments may not have launched vaccination programs, it is clear that the principal medical journals of the era were unqualified in their support for Jenner's methods. Some physicians offered testimonials of their own successful use of Jenner's methods. Many made an additional contribution by rebutting William Goldson's conclusions that the protection provided was only very temporary.

For example, in the *Philadelphia Medical Museum* several physicians offered a direct rebuttal to the pamphlet published by vaccination skeptic William Goldson in 1804. One contributor was fairly measured in their response, conceding that permanent immunization had not yet been proven—after all, the vaccine had been introduced just a decade earlier. But still, the writer argued, the evidence clearly suggested that the vaccine was providing complete protection thus far. Moreover, most of the supposed cases of smallpox occurring among vaccinated populations could be explained either as something other than smallpox or due to the failure of the initial vaccination to actually take. Possibly, inexperienced administers had failed to recognize that their procedure produced only a local rather than a systemic response. Dr. John Church was less conciliatory in rebutting Goldson. Goldson was far too willing to spread conclusions drawn from shoddy research, Church argued, proof that his purpose was to "to disturb the peaceful interests of society." And the journal editor was even more harsh in condemning local practitioners who questioned vaccination. They simply saw greater profits in inoculation and preyed on the poor and needy.[37]

Other contributors took a more positive approach, asserting the evidence of vaccination's effectiveness. John Redman Coxe offered the example of his own son—Edward Jenner Coxe—as proof that the vaccine worked. He had treated the child when only nine days old, and subsequently had intentionally exposed his son to smallpox three times before he reached the age of four. (Despite his father's experimental zeal, the child did live to see his fifth birthday.) A report from the French minister of the interior published in the *Philadelphia Medical and Physical Journal* demonstrated a similar reckless enthusiasm. He reported that six Black children vaccinated on the Isle de Bourbon had provided the material used to vaccinate five thousand other people. And like Coxe's test subject, the children were repeatedly exposed to smallpox to demonstrate the efficacy of the procedure.[38]

These medical journals also published a carrot-and-stick approach to encouraging vaccination. While a medical society in Lausanne was offering 1,000 livres to anyone who contracted smallpox after being vaccinated, the Royal Jennerian Society emphasized the danger of refusing vaccination. In the half-century before Jenner's discovery more than 100,000 people had died from smallpox—or about 2,000 annually—in Great Britain. But in 1804 only 586 British residents had fallen to the disease.[39]

By 1805 Dr. John Spence was reporting in the *Medical Museum* that the public relations campaign was paying off. Goldson's pamphlet might have produced a "clamor" when initially released, but just a year later more and more people were coming to accept the safety and value of vaccination. During a recent outbreak in Dumfries, Virginia, even slaves were asking to be vaccinated, he reported. And individuals previously vaccinated were taking "advantage of the opportunity" to expose themselves to the disease to prove their invincibility.[40]

The humanitarian motivations of these vaccination crusaders are undeniable. But they must also have recognized that smallpox vaccination promised to boost the prestige of their profession. It was clearly the most significant, impressive achievement of medical science in decades—a safer and less taxing answer to one of the century's great killers. And no doubt doctors also envisioned the ancillary benefits for medical science that would follow vaccination's wider acceptance. Convincing the public that vaccination was just the first victory—believing that left unfettered, physicians might conquer other ailments and diseases—physicians pleaded with the public to surrender more corpses for dissection. More than one contributor closed their account of a fatal illness by suggesting that dissection of the corpse would have helped them understand the illness—and increased their ability to properly treat patients in the future.

Yet for all these physicians' interest in advancing the prestige of the profession and increasing public confidence in medicine, it is clear that the public remained unconvinced. Testimonials to the efficacy of medicine's most impressive achievement were surrounded in these journals by stories of patient resistance, accounts of the sick and wounded choosing to follow their own counsel despite the celebratory claims of physicians trumpeting the growing dominion of medical science over disease. And in truth, while the achievements of medical science were one of the recurring refrains in these journals, contributing physicians could be surprisingly humble in acknowledging persistent limitations in the current science. Revealing that theirs was less a coherent campaign than professional wish, they coupled their calls for more confidence in their methods, more latitude in their research, and greater compliance from their patients with surprising humility in acknowledging their own diagnostic errors. A Dr. Harris admitted that they failed to recognize the signs of hydrocephalus which killed their young patient. Not only had they fatally misread this particular case; they now suspected there were "several cases in which I might have overlooked the disease." And William Dewees, though not really the sort to publicize his own faults, was willing to point out the errors of his colleagues. After discovering mid-delivery that a baby had passed through a rupture in the uterus and had to be extricated from the mother's intestines, he acknowledged that the pelvic abnormality that caused the rupture, and the death of the mother and child, could have and should have been discovered through a routine examination.[41]

In the twenty years following the yellow fever crisis, important steps were taken to establish some sort of consensus around disease. Under Elihu Hubbard Smith's direction the *Medical Repository* launched a campaign to build orthodoxy, defend Benjamin Rush, and defang his critics. For decades the journal was uncompromising and uncritical in promoting one all-encompassing explanation for disease. Other journals were less narrowly partisan—still, they were as unfocused as they were inclusive.

But while the *Repository* might have thus succeeded in dominating the professional playing field and maintaining a more sustained and authoritative position within professional discourse, it did not enjoy anything close to unquestioned authority among the general public. Laypeople—the physicians' patients—remained resistant to their demands, suspicious of their methods, and skeptical of their prescriptions. Laypeople reached their own conclusions and offered their own theories; they resisted the recommendations of physicians and occasionally bullied their doctors into therapies the professionals questioned. Armed with self-help manuals and reassured by pantries filled with patent medicines, the American public was not ready to surrender the medical playing field to the doctors.

And it is this stubborn independence of the public on questions of health and therapeutics that must be acknowledged in understanding—even sharing blame for—the stagnation of American disease theory in the nineteenth century. While Smith and the *Repository* worked to canonize a specific mode of analysis and treatment, it seems clear that large portions of the public inclined toward these same conclusions—that they clung to the same ancient theories of miasmatic origins and, especially in the wake of the 1793 yellow fever epidemic, depended on the heroic therapies they believed most likely to protect them.

There is plenty of evidence to suggest that during the 1793 epidemic public opinion tended to side with Rush—that as the crisis progressed, a large portion, perhaps most, of the general public fell into Rush's camp. Judge William Bradford proclaimed Rush the "darling of the common people," and Rush himself seemed to think that the public was on his side. His letters repeatedly referenced the public demand for his time and treatments—the parents "weeping aloud for me, all calling upon me to hasten to the relief of their sick." He also claimed that his purging powder grew in popularity as the epidemic progressed. In fact, based on testimonials and advertisements in the papers, he might have been correct.[42]

But all this only begs the real question: Why would the general public embrace Rush's theory of yellow fever's miasmatic origins and submit to his draconian therapies?

For more than a half-century many scholars have embraced the idea that, at least in Europe, ideological and economic factors informed the responses of physicians and lay commentators to etiological questions. Predominantly liberal and bourgeoise, they leaned toward an explanation of disease that did not imply the need for restrictions on travel and trade. Better to blame local filth and throw their weight behind civic-minded sanitation measures than endorse contagionist ideas that would lead to quarantines and blockades.[43]

Some historians have challenged this argument, finding "no correlation between anti-contagionism and politics in America." Nineteenth-century medical writers cited a range of considerations in rebutting contagionist ideas—science, religion, even appeals to motherhood—but at bottom, they based their arguments on "strictly medical grounds." Influenced by neither politics nor economics, "independent medical opinion" lay behind the widespread preference for miasmatic over contagionist theories.[44]

It is an argument that becomes even more persuasive when we recall where we began: with an appreciation for the fact that during this period disease was "a sensory experience, filled with distinctive sights, smells, and sounds." Contagionist arguments struggled because they could not identify, describe, or really even conceive of the thing that was being transferred from person to person. Without any understanding of bacteria or viruses, unable to link their ideas to any broader appreciation for the micro-organisms we recognize as fundamental to biology, contagionists were forced to root their ideas in something invisible and undetectable. Rush and his followers, on the other hand, could point to the proof offered by the senses—the foul odor wafting from the putrefying carcass, the nauseating stench emanating from the rotting garbage, the actually visible miasma lifting from the stagnant, crust-covered pond. These ideas met with popular approval because they squared with what early Americans found so plausible, that illness and its causes could be smelled, seen, and even tasted. This was plausible because it was tied to even more fundamental confidences in both the reliability of human senses and the decipherability of God's universe. Miasmatic theories were democratic, resting on the premise, as one historian has argued, that "one's self was a good guide to the qualities of an environment," and buttressed by the cosmological confidences of post-Calvinist Protestantism—a "widespread faith that the world spoke in signs that all were equipped to interpret."[45]

But while these fundamental understandings of disease might explain the relative popularity of Rush's miasmatic theories, it is still surprising that his body-wrenching course of treatment would be so widely embraced. Why would yellow fever victims spurn more mild treatments and submit to his painful and debilitating therapies, which placed far greater demands on the body? And if, as Rush's critics both then and now have argued, his therapies were ineffective, why did so many swear otherwise?

Part of the answer might lie in the confidence with which Rush trumpeted his success. He boasted that better than 90 percent of those he purged and bled did not succumb to yellow fever. And, in a certain sense, this may have been true. He urged patients to seek treatment at the first sign of sickness—an aching head, throat, or back; nausea; chills. Purging and bleeding on the first day, in the first hour, were essential, he stressed, for recovery, and consequently no doubt many underwent treatment for nothing worse than a mild cold or poor night's sleep. Many of Rush's critics suggested as much, but Rush and his supporters countered with an unanswerable demand for proof that Rush's patients had not been infected with the fever. Meanwhile, those undergoing treatment, thrilled that their symptoms never worsened, gratefully joined the celebratory chorus.

And a nervous public, anxious to believe that a cure was available, leapt at the good news.[46]

But the testimonials offered in support of Rush's treatment did far more than declare its effectiveness—they suggested that there was something appealing in Rush's heroic approach, something attractive in the very violence of its methods and the graphic nature of its effects.

Rush's patients paid tribute to the doctor by describing their symptoms and treatments in vivid detail; they boasted of the ounces of blood taken, the number of stools passed, the color and texture of the vomit puked. One grateful supporter published his tribute to Rush in verse:

> Within the stomach humours did convene,
> And vomiting did often supervene;
> The bile was black, and putrid too indeed
> And hemorrhages sometimes did succeed. . . .
>
> The eyes grew red, their pupils did dilate;
> The fluids rush'd into a putrid state,
> The thirst was great, the urine color'd high;
> The tongue turn'd white, the skin was hot and dry. . . .
>
> The celebrated Dr. Rush did find,
> That calomel, with jalap well combin'd,
> Was the best purge, by far, that could be giv'n. . . .
>
> Evacuations of these kinds repressed
> The raging plague and thus sav'd the distress'd.[47]

Rush's fans were not the only ones to offer up colorful accounts of their illness; his critics were as ready as his supporters to color their analysis with graphic detail. In fact, in providing the gory details, the unfiltered descriptions of the sights, sounds, and smells of illness, these victims were in part simply embracing a common form of medical discourse. After all, this was a world in which health and illness could only be measured by the sensed. With no understanding of the microscopic agents to which we immediately turn today in diagnosing and treating disease, graphic details lay at the heart of contemporary etiology. Therefore, laypeople provided richly detailed accounts of their experiences just as physicians on both sides of the debate laced their arguments and advice with graphic descriptions of the symptoms to expect and monitor.[48]

But within the graphic accounts provided by Rush's supporters, one also senses a certain pride in their gory combat, a belief that there was something telling, even praiseworthy, in their victory over the disease, and within this the hint that they chose Rush's aggressive therapeutics because they liked the idea that their recovery depended on their submission to, or better, endurance of heroic measures. For his part, Rush liked to emphasize that his treatments could be tolerated by virtually everyone. He noted that Margaret Meredith, wife of US treasurer Samuel Meredith, successfully took his purge, "even though a woman of uncommon delicacy of constitution." But his patients preferred to stress the severity of the treatments and, implicitly, their own fortitude in tolerating them. In a letter to the *Federal Gazette* George Hunter boasted that several members of his family, ranging in age from four to seventy-three, endured both the fever's "violence of symptoms" and the equally violent but effective countermeasures. Rush bled some of his relatives, Hunter crowed, as many as five times. Another correspondent noted that Dr. John Pennington's road to recovery covered five bleedings and an impressively "liberal use of the mercurial powders." The war story of another grateful patient also emphasized the violent pain that racked his body, as well as the "copious bleeding" that saved him from the grave. And Dr. Samuel Griffitts encouraged victims to not fear the lancet within a thinly veiled celebration of his own courage and strength: "If my poor frame, reduced by previous sickness, great anxiety, and fatigue, and a very low diet, could bear seven bleedings in five days, besides purging and no diet but toast and water, what shall we say to physicians who bleed but once."[49]

In other words, Rush's treatment allowed patients to tell themselves, and others, that they had wrestled the disease into submission through a body-wrenching program, not simply waited it out through a gentle regimen of cool baths and quinine. In addition to this ego-massaging reward, Rush's rugged therapy might have been appealing because, in a certain sense, it actually worked. It may not have cured—but it worked in that it forced a powerful response from the body. Unlike cool baths, soothing drinks, and most of all patience—advice that for patients and their desperate families might have been simply too passive, an unsatisfying invitation to death—Rush's purging powders caused the bowels to explode while his lancets calmed the pulse and quieted victims wracked with pain and made delirious by fever. And in forcing these responses from the body, Rush suggested that he enjoyed some mastery over it. In turn, when patients came out on the other side and celebrated their own ability to endure the treatment, to survive copious bleedings and violent evacuations, they celebrated their own mastery over their bodies as well.[50]

Reviewing the "currents and counter-currents in medical science" for the Massachusetts Medical Society in 1860, Oliver Wendell Holmes acknowledged Rush's extraordinary influence: "He taught thousands of American students, he gave a direction to the medical mind of the country more than any other one man." But this was cause for regret, Holmes said, as Rush embodied many unfortunate "tendencies of the American medical mind, its self-confidence, its audacious handling of Nature, its impatience with her old-fashioned ways of taking time to get a sick man well." But Holmes also conceded that Rush's etiological and therapeutic systems were fully in sync with American sensibilities:

> How could a people which has a revolution once in four years, which has contrived the Bowie-knife and the revolver, which has chewed the juice out of all the superlatives in the language in Fourth of July orations, . . . which insists in sending out yachts and horses and boys to out-sail, out-run, out-fight, and checkmate all the rest of creation; how could such a people be content with any but "heroic" practice? What wonder that the stars and stripes wave over doses of ninety grains of sulphate of quinine, . . . and that the American eagle screams with delight to see three drachms of calomel given at a single mouthful?

Holmes placed a particular emphasis on the Revolution as a formative experience for Rush and his followers. "His own mind was in a perpetual state of exaltation produced by the stirring scenes in which he had taken a part," Holmes explained. "He could not help feeling as if Nature had been a good deal shaken by the Declaration of Independence, and that American art was getting to be rather too much for her."[51] But in truth, a good deal of Rush's medical philosophy, and that of the public which embraced his ideas, can be traced to additional sources—the sensory-based physiology of John Brown, the proliferation of the medicines and literature of medical self-management. And one critical component within this approach to health and disease—the emphasis on self-mastery that is the corollary of heroic therapy—had even deeper roots in American culture. Puritans suggested that it could offer proof of one's salvation; republicans argued that controlling one's ambitions and subordinating one's private interests to the welfare of the community were essential to good government.

As a result, this constellation of ideas about disease and therapy, rooted in ancient concepts, central elements of American culture, new science, and emerging features of the medical marketplace, acquired a new vitality in the years after the 1793 epidemic. Both laypeople and professionals tapped into the prevailing belief that health and disease remained sensory experiences—that the body was acutely sensitive to its surroundings, that the threats to it were readily detectable by our senses, and that the most effective therapies could be witnessed as they did their curative, albeit violent, work. A physician could identify the threats to his patients through an assessment of environmental conditions—the purity of the air that they breathed, the cleanliness of the water that they tasted, the amount of putrefaction they could see and smell—and patients could gauge the efficacy of a treatment by the trauma it forced on their bodies and the degree of fortitude it took to endure it.

It would have made Benjamin Rush and his literary apologist Elihu Smith proud to know that when Americans confronted their next medical crisis, they brought to the challenge much the same analysis that framed their response to the epidemics of the 1790s. Less satisfying to Rush and Smith would have been the reaction of both professionals and laypeople when this analysis proved inadequate. As these ideas about local miasmas and heroic therapies proved unable to explain or address the crisis presented by cholera in 1832, Americans—both professional and lay—questioned key pieces of their medical philosophy, and perhaps most importantly, the reliability of the senses on which they had come to rely.

6

Cholera and the Emergence of the Gothic in American Medical Culture

IN 1831 AMERICANS WATCHED nervously as cholera swept westward across the European continent. Natural and human barriers seemed unable to slow the disease as it crossed mountains, rivers, and military cordons. As Americans considered the real possibility that the epidemic might leap the Atlantic, many must have thought back to the 1790s and the yellow fever epidemics that had plagued American cities in that decade. True, the medical landscape had evolved somewhat since then. There were more medical schools, and several cities had launched sanitation projects aimed at reducing the filth in and adjacent to urban centers. And as we will see in the next chapter, a host of "irregular" practitioners offered systems and cures that challenged regular physicians. But at the heart of medical practice the same set of ideas about putrefaction and toxic effluvia still dominated disease theory. And so as American physicians confronted their second health crisis since the War for Independence, they brought little new in the way of explanation or treatment.

There was, however, one significant difference: As this new crisis wore on, many expressed less patience with old formulas—physicians voiced less confidence in their ability to unravel and treat the escalating medical threat, while laypeople resorted to dark, fatalistic lamentations about the creeping menace that seemed beyond all human powers to intercept and defeat. In 1793 Rush and his followers had expressed confidence that more and more disease was falling under the dominion of medical science, but by 1833 pessimism surrounding the latest failure of medicine had soured public attitudes and chastened professional ambitions.

"Cholera" was not an unknown disease to Americans in 1830.[1] They had dealt with their own version of this disease frequently before. Usually referred to as "cholera morbus," this more mild and manageable intestinal disorder was a recurring visitor to American communities. But reports filling European press through the 1820s made clear that the plague assaulting Europe was different. This "Asiatic" or "spasmodic" cholera was both more deadly and more painful. A bacterial infection that rapidly reproduces in the small intestine, the disease yields severe diarrhea and consequently dehydration and the loss of critical minerals. If untreated, death occurs in more than half the cases.[2]

In 1849 an English physician, John Snow, identified a public water pump as the source of a cholera outbreak in London; later in the century researchers would conclude that the disease was transmitted through cholera victims' feces that made their way into water supplies. But in 1830, without this knowledge, Americans were left struck by cholera's virulence and, more frighteningly, its incredible mobility. Previously, British and American sources had viewed Asiatic cholera as an East Indian disease—a deadly part of the exotic country—and described it with the mixture of horror and curiosity that distance allowed. But as the killer began its march westward in 1817, this sense of safety disappeared. A contributor to the *Daily National Intelligencer*, recounting the progress of the disease over the preceding decade, observed that it became more malignant as it spread. Formerly only a "mild climatic disease," it was claiming thousands of lives and advancing fifteen miles a day, moving from east to west across the breadth of India in just twelve months. The epidemic also moved east, leaping across seas to attack islands off the Indochina peninsula. But its more dangerous path was to the West. Following routes carved by travel and trade, it soon reached the Persian Gulf. By the time it reached the southern Russian city of Astrakhan, the disease had killed sixty thousand people.[3] Handkerchiefs soaked in camphor were no match for the cholera that poured through the city "like a mountain torrent" before setting off across the heart of Russia on the currents of the Volga.[4]

The interest of the American press in the disease increased with each new country it infected. But Americans also benefited from the knowledge gained by those on the frontlines. By the time cholera reached Western Europe, medical and civic officials could draw on the experience of Eastern Europeans—and for those already hit by the disease this direct experience had been educative.[5] A large literature focused primarily on the question of transmissibility had emerged as the disease spread through Russia, Poland, Austria, and Prussia. Medical professionals in Russia were the first to conclude that the disease was not contagious—that it was not transmitted from person to person.[6] This does not mean that the lay response was either calm or grounded in science. Despite the conclusions reached by medical professionals, public officials in Russia, Germany, and Poland tended to take a better-safe-than-sorry approach and recommended remarkably severe restrictions on travel and trade. The autocratic structure of these governments made implementation possible. In Prussia sixty thousand troops were dispatched to the eastern border. Stationed at one-hundred-yard intervals and reenforced by cavalry units, the troops cordoned off the country from all travel and trade. Even those permitted to cross the border had their possessions, including their money and letters, fumigated. Individual towns imposed their own preventative measures. Persons displaying suspicious symptoms were forced into hospitals where they were stripped and scrubbed—externally with chloride of lime and internally with harsh purgatives like calomel. Diseased houses were emptied, the owners forced to surrender keys while their doors and windows were nailed shut. Even the dogs and cats roaming the village streets fell under suspicion and consequently were rounded up and killed.[7]

The measures were not accepted without complaint and in places met outright resistance, especially by the poor. They balked at the newly mandated burial practices that forbade traditional opportunities for mourning and protested the commercial restrictions that cost them affordable goods and often jobs. And on these economic issues they found allies in merchants and shopkeepers.[8]

This resistance was assisted by the emerging consensus that cholera was not contagious. To prove the point one Prussian doctor thrust his hand into the cadaver of a recent victim and climbed naked into the bed of the dying. Instead, a growing number of doctors argued that the disease was rooted in putrefaction and filth, and preyed most opportunistically on the intemperate and those compromised by poor diets and hygiene. By late 1831 this analysis provided the autocratic governments of Eastern Europe with the medical basis needed to justify their retreat from their earlier coercive measures. Moved by the anti-contagionist arguments, unsettled by protests from the unlikely alliance of merchants and the poor, and struggling with the practical tasks of policing lengthy borders, these governments abandoned or significantly tempered their earlier measures.[9]

Western Europeans tracked the evolving response and, while still safely removed, seemed to accept the growing anti-contagion consensus. But once cholera reached their own borders, this calm dissipated. France quickly dispatched thirty thousand soldiers to its northern and eastern borders. The response in Britain was more restrained, but still the Royal College of Physicians concluded that the disease might be spread by goods, leading the London Board of Health to impose a temporary quarantine on imported articles.[10]

Yet the panic faded more quickly in the West than the East. Too much evidence of cholera's noncontagious character had been gathered—and so the resistance to these measures by merchants and a large sector of the medical community grew quickly. In France this opposition was led by Nicolas Chervin. The University of Paris–trained physician had traveled broadly researching yellow fever, concluding that the contagionist theories surrounding the disease and the quarantines these inspired were misguided. Now he staked out a similar position on cholera, and his conclusions were incorporated in a report from the Academies of Medicine and Science that was skeptical of human-to-human transmission and flat out denied the transportability of the disease via goods. In Britain, Charles Maclean, physician and longtime employee of the East India Company, continued the campaign against contagionism and quarantines that he had launched in the previous decade. He drew on the miasmatic theories he had defended for years and condemned quarantines as not only economically foolish but immoral, as they resulted in the healthy abandoning the sick.[11]

American commentators similarly benefited from the lessons learned in Europe. In particular, early reports glommed onto analyses that afforded some rationality or predictability to the disease. Washington, D.C.'s *Daily National Journal* printed a Polish account that suggested the disease was the concomitant of war and would persist only so long as the war with Russia continued.[12] The Washington *Globe* quoted a Russian observer who noted that the disease was preceded by the appearance of "dense masses of small green flies"—a recurring feature of Asian epidemics.[13] But the most common analysis emphasized the disease's primary targets: The most vulnerable, it was argued, were the poor and intemperate. While those leading sober, disciplined lives were largely insulated from the disease, persons who lived in filth; who resided in crowded, poorly ventilated neighborhoods; and who failed to lead lives of regularity—in diet, drink, and sex—were the only ones really at risk.[14] This analysis was given a different edge in an account printed in the *Boston Courier* in April 1832. Not only were the poor the most susceptible but their resistance to defensive public measures compounded their vulnerability. A father who refused to turn his child over to authorities for burial was singled out as representative of the "barbarous conduct" that left poor neighborhoods at heightened risk for infection.[15]

This message, reassuring to many, did not go unchallenged, however. In particular, a growing body of evidence suggested that the disease was far less selective. A letter from a private citizen in Hamburg, printed in the *United States' Telegraph* in November 1831, reported that contrary to some published accounts, "persons of the higher class"—bankers and merchants—were falling to the disease.[16] And these accounts of the disease's indiscriminate reach were coupled with a growing recognition that cholera's noncontagious character was not necessarily good news. If not spread through person-to-person contact, how was it spreading? In what mysterious way had the disease managed to cover so much ground in such little time?

When cholera jumped the Atlantic and reached Canada in June 1832, these more troubling accounts fed a growing hysteria in the United States. The dreaded disease "may now be daily expected among us," warned the *Daily National Intelligencer*.[17] In part to defuse the growing alarm, Philadelphia officials dispatched a medical commission to study the epidemics attacking Quebec and Montreal.

The conclusions the commission reached offered cause for concern. Cholera's mobility was astounding. After reaching Quebec in early June, the disease traveled some six hundred miles along the Saint Lawrence Seaway in just twenty days. But the commission's findings in Quebec also offered a reassuring message. Those most immediately affected were the emigrants crowding the low-lying neighborhoods surrounding the docks. They were bound for the interior, but before setting off they lived in crowded quarters, ate poor food, were prone to intemperance, and subject to other diseases associated with squalid conditions like typhus.[18]

In Montreal, the commission reached some different but equally reassuring conclusions. The emigrant population seemed to be less susceptible to infection than natives. But a set of local conditions were blamed for the spread of the disease. A sluggish stream running through a ravine in the center of town had become the repository for all sorts of garbage and filth. A tell-tale putrid odor issued from the mucky creek, evidence of the sort of toxic miasma Philadelphia physicians had linked to epidemic disease for decades. It was no surprise, they concluded, that 90 percent of the cholera cases were situated in close proximity to this ravine.[19]

The message coming from the Philadelphia commission was clear: While the triggering conditions varied, the epidemic in both cities was due largely to the failure of civic officials to take any sort of measures to protect residents from the malevolent miasmas that had plagued people for centuries. Streets had not been cleaned; swamps and gullies had not been drained; hospitals had not been established. In fact, these failures actually fed the panic that swept through the city, and this panic, "acting on the systems of hundreds already laboring under the universal predisposition which is observed to influence a community during the prevalence of the epidemic," actually increased the public's susceptibility to the disease. In other words, had appropriate public measures been imposed quickly, at the earliest signs of cholera's arrival, much of the crisis might have been averted.[20]

Philadelphia was not the only city to investigate the disease. Once cholera hit American soil, the New York Board of Health asked for a report from the city's physicians as well as for them to collect information from other cities and towns. And to a certain extent the information gathered echoed the reassuring message of the Philadelphia commission. New York's hospital physicians concluded that the disease fell "in a remarkable degree upon the dissolute and intemperate"; "drunks and prostitutes" represented a majority of the victims. The doctors conceded that a few cases did not fit within this category, but these could be traced to some "act of gross imprudence." For example, a father and his three children succumbed to cholera after bingeing on berries and milk.[21]

The same report also concluded, like the Philadelphia commission, that the disease was probably not contagious. It could not be traced to some arriving vessel; it tended to occur in low-lying, swampy neighborhoods, and its rapid spread suggested it traveled by air. The various elements of their analysis were summarized in their conclusion that the "low Irish" suffered most. They were intemperate, "dirty in their habits," and lived in squalid basement apartments. A report from the hospital on Rivington Street similarly pointed the finger at the city's Irish residents. They were poor; lived in filthy, crowded homes; and were "daily intoxicated." The report did concede that many hard-working women were among the early victims. But while not guilty of intemperance, they were broken down by their labor and thus more vulnerable to disease than their more affluent neighbors.[22]

Reports from the surrounding towns offered similar conclusions. A doctor in Troy found no evidence of contagion, no evidence of a foreign source, and fatal cases confined to the poor, dirty, and intemperate. A Dr. Dubois of New Utrecht found much the same.[23] Yet as the epidemic persisted, more people began to question the tidiness of these early analyses. After the New York Board of Health suggested that the specifics of the epidemic rendered any sort of quarantine unnecessary as it would only stifle commerce and increase unemployment, a writer to the *Daily National Intelligencer* attacked the conclusions of this "self-constituted body." And this was followed by J. R. Rhinelander, a member of the board, resigning in protest because more damaging reports had been "suppressed, the facts bent to suit particular opinions and object."[24] A team of doctors sent to New York from Providence to investigate the epidemic joined this dissent. They argued that in suggesting that only the intemperate and unclean were susceptible to the disease, the Special Medical Council had inhibited doctors from reporting cases that did not fit this conclusion. In reality, the death toll from the disease was "FRIGHTFULLY GREAT." After documenting more than two hundred cases, they declared, "Death seemed to Ride Triumphant and govern with almost despotic sway."[25]

After anxiously watching this disease cross continents and oceans, the public must have been unsettled by these more alarming reports. And people closely reading the Philadelphia commissioners' report must also have been struck by their even more unnerving confession. Beneath their rosy prediction that individuals leading temperate and comfortable lives would be safe lay the admission that the deeper nature of the disease—its origins, root cause, and means of transmission—were unknown, and quite possibly would never be known. In the sort of admission that would never have been made within the intellectual climate of 1793, these physicians conceded that "it may not be within the limited power of our very finite capacities to ascertain the natural causes in the action of which pestilential diseases originate." Nor did they believe further research might prove useful. In fact, the epidemic had already inspired a voluminous literature. But the lack of consensus within it only offered proof that all observations were "equally conjectural" and the fundamental questions still rooted in "obscurity and ignorance." Starkly put, the potential for human efforts to "penetrate the nature of final causes" would be limited by the "finite power of our senses."[26]

The great systematizers of the preceding century were never so pessimistic. They may have differed on root causes, but they believed those causes existed and would ultimately be brought under the dominion of medical science. This investigative team was more sober in assessing its ability to understand the root of disease, as well as the therapeutic tools that might bring disease under human control. The best that might be hoped for was some limited understanding of the laws that guide its growth and expansion. Communities facing deadly outbreaks might hope at best to "control their energy, [and] restrict the extent of their prevalence."[27] Rush, who followed his announcement that he had found a cure for yellow fever with the prediction that soon all other diseases, including the plague, would be brought under the power of medicine, no doubt turned over in his grave.

Even the conclusions the commission did reach about the general nature of epidemics were far from encouraging. The report suggested that no disease would reach epidemic proportions unless there also existed an "epidemic influence"—some set of conditions that enabled a specific ailment to afflict a community with particular mortality. Moreover, these epidemic "influences or constitutions" seemed to recur at certain disease-specific intervals. For example, yellow fever had spread within a particular atmospheric constitution from 1793 to 1805. But the duration of these periods and their intervals were a mystery.[28]

Even more troubling, these "influences or constitutions" were not the disease itself—not the discrete ailment that might through some investigatory process yield clues to its eradication—but rather some set of obscure and still mysterious atmospheric, climatic, and/or terrestrial conditions that acted on humans, compromising their ability to resist or manage what were at other times less terrible diseases. The very indecipherability of these epidemic influences that weakened "certain organs and ... certain functions of the economy" meant that the outlook for communities awaiting the arrival of cholera was grim.[29] They were not placed at risk by a discrete morbid substance; their safety could not be assured by a rigorous campaign of isolation, fumigation, quarantine, or sanitation. They were under some sort of mysterious cosmological assault, their bodies being targeted by an unidentifiable atmospheric or terrestrial condition that left them weak and vulnerable to diseases that might at other times be manageable.

It should be noted that this emphasis on epidemic influences or constitutions was not entirely new. In his 1799 *Brief History of Epidemic and Pestilential Diseases,* Noah Webster expanded on the theory introduced by

Hippocrates and developed more recently by Sydenham that some alteration of the atmosphere transformed a relatively manageable local miasma into a more deadly epidemical toxin. Webster went further, coupling this conclusion to an extensive exploration of the possible sources of this atmospheric change. Noting that epidemics almost always coincided, at least loosely, with some violent temporal convulsion—earthquakes, volcanos, severe droughts, harsh winters—he suggested that the planets might exert some influence on the atmosphere based on "the great laws of attraction and repulsion." Webster similarly drew on a wide body of literature to methodically explore the relationship—either causal or predictive—among comets, earthquakes, the weather, and human health.[30]

Moreover, Webster's conclusion was embraced enthusiastically by Rush and others, like Charles Caldwell, Rush's former student, investigating the disease at the tail end of the century. Rush described these revelations as yet another "mine of precious metals to the lovers of science"—affirmation of his own long-held suspicion that "the malignant constitution of the atmosphere" was yet another contributing factor to the spread of disease.[31]

But whereas Rush had greeted Webster's 1799 discovery with excitement, viewing it as yet another piece in the puzzle that would lead to the eventual eradication of disease, those referencing these mysterious disturbances of the cosmos during the 1832 cholera epidemic were far less ambitious in exploring their character and far less hopeful as to where all this would lead. The Philadelphia commission was thorough in its description of the medical symptoms that indicated the existence of an epidemic constitution but conspicuously silent on the possible causes of this atmospheric anomaly. Instead, their reference to these mysterious atmospheric convulsions was embedded within the same pessimistic assessment of humankind's ability to unravel the larger mystery of disease.

And other observers—laypeople contributing analyses to the press—were even less likely to tie their references to these threatening atmospheric conditions to any sort of scientific speculation, instead embedding them within forecasts that were eerily sinister. A report in the *New-York Spectator* concluded that the disease's origins were "atmospheric," apparently crossing the Atlantic on easterly winds that blew for a portentous forty days.³² Another tickled biblical memories of Mosaic visitations with the suggestion that the skies were filled with "myriads of insects too small for detection by the naked eye," producing "an unwholesome state of the atmosphere."³³ And the gloom within these forecasts resonated with a darker portrait of disease that had gathered strength as cholera made its way across Europe and North America. As the disease scaled mountains and crossed oceans, as quarantines and sanitary cordons proved ineffective, a portion of the public response grew dark, even gothic—characterized by horror and a fatalistic acceptance of, and at times indulgence in, the inevitable crisis. Writers obsessed on the morbid details of the illness and the hopeless and gruesome suffering of its victims. Finding no comfort in science or government, these gothic accounts described a mysterious killer, an infectious and irresistible cloud, capable of crossing vast swatches of geography at alarming speeds.³⁴

Historians have described the emergence of gothic styles and themes within the murder and crime narratives of the early republic and Americans' concomitant growing fascination with horror. This shift within literary style, and more broadly the perceptions of crime and criminals, went hand in hand with the erosion of the "sacred master plot." As people lost confidence in traditional religious explanations—as they were no longer content to simply attribute violence and crime to the persistence of evil in the world—they embraced a new literature and new explanation that focused more on the individual details of crimes and criminals. Murder narratives now concentrated on the gruesome details of the crime and the daily habits of the criminal in a search for the specific factors at play: the motives, the unleashed passions, or the environmental influences that led a person to a specific criminal act.³⁵

This more complex exploration of violence resonated with the Enlightenment confidence of the era—the search for motives was tied to the belief that the natural world was not a battleground between the forces of good and evil but instead a place inhabited by humans who were ultimately reasonable, a place where even bad behavior could be explained. But as the nineteenth century advanced, more and more of these narratives failed to reach satisfying conclusions. Too many horrific crimes could not be explained through rational analysis, and too many murders could not be reconciled with the Enlightenment's positive view of human nature. As a result, many crimes were portrayed as simply incomprehensible and the killer cast as a monster, an aberration, an inhuman beast. These crimes were no longer portrayed as illustrations of the sin within us all but rather as a reminder that the universe still contained aspects that could be neither understood nor imagined.

These increasingly popular crime narratives of the first half of the nineteenth century shared much with the emerging gothic fiction in which the villain was cast as incomprehensibly dark. And both genres exhibited a growing fascination with the details of the grisly deeds done by these inhuman beasts. Crime narratives and gothic tales indulged in a gory recitation of the murderous acts, the weapons, the wounds, and the blood-splattered scenes. One historian suggests this fascination constituted a "pornography of violence," a self-conscious indulgence that can only be understood within the context of expanding humanitarian values. As people embraced the values of refinement and sympathy, as they came to see suffering and pain not as some inevitable part of life but something that could and should be avoided, as they questioned the appropriateness of everything from blood sports to vivisection, they turned to a literature of violence as a sort of "dreadful pleasure."[36]

There is much within the popular reaction to the cholera epidemic that resonates with the styles and themes of this growing literature of crime and violence, as well as the tropes of gothic literature. As early as August 1831, before rumors of the disease reaching England were confirmed, observers speculated that the disease would sneak past government measures and "creep in, in some way or other."[37] Cholera did not follow any logical course; it traveled in "a mysterious manner," driven by causes "entirely unknown."[38] Challenging the assertions of science, exposing the false confidences of medicine, one writer eventually concluded that the disease would soon spread over the whole American continent, "as it seems to be governed by no fixed laws."[39] This characterization of the disease as a "creeping" menace was often coupled to imagery of the illness as a toxic cloud or wave. One writer mocked a simpleton overheard arguing that the black spot on the sun was not Jupiter passing between the earth and the sun but rather "the cholera . . . on its way from Russia and Poland to New Orleans."[40] But the simpleton found more than a few serious supporters who likened the disease to some malevolent force, smothering all in its path "as if the vials of Eternal Wrath had been poured out upon them by the terrible angel of the pestilence."[41] The identity of this gothic killer took different forms—one called it "the insatiate destroyer," another the "Destroying Angel."[42] Yet common to all was the fact of cholera's irresistible power. Now that the formless killer had "broken through all quarantine barriers," one observer lamented, little remained but "fear, sorrow, misery, and death."[43] Even the science-minded medical commission appointed to investigate the Canadian epidemics had noted that the disease "burst" on the cities "as though pestilence had rained down on them from an impending cloud."[44]

In some accounts, as cholera took on a character, a persona, it acquired the power to kill by terror alone. The *Cherokee Phoenix* reported an experiment in St. Petersburg in which condemned criminals were quartered in a hospital room previously occupied by cholera victims, even sleeping in the same beds. Not told about the prior occupants, inmates emerged from the experience with their health intact. Once transferred, however, to a clean, sanitary room, one untouched by the disease, and then falsely told that their current quarters had previously housed cholera patients, four of the six died within days.[45]

As these gothic accounts of the disease spread, so too did the quantitative hyperbole. One writer estimated that over the previous fourteen years, cholera had killed 50 million people, decimating three continents.[46] Another anticipated a common gothic literary device in reporting the horror of one cholera victim being mistakenly buried alive. Even when observers noted several chest spasms, he was "thrust into his narrow home."[47]

Just as writers painted a gothic portrait of the disease, they indulged in graphic portraits of the victims that resembled the popular literature of horror. A victim described the horrible agony—his stomach "as if it contained a furnace. The thirst was unslakable . . . intolerable cramps that threatened to tear him to pieces."[48] One recovering victim declared that, so horrific were the symptoms, should the disease return,

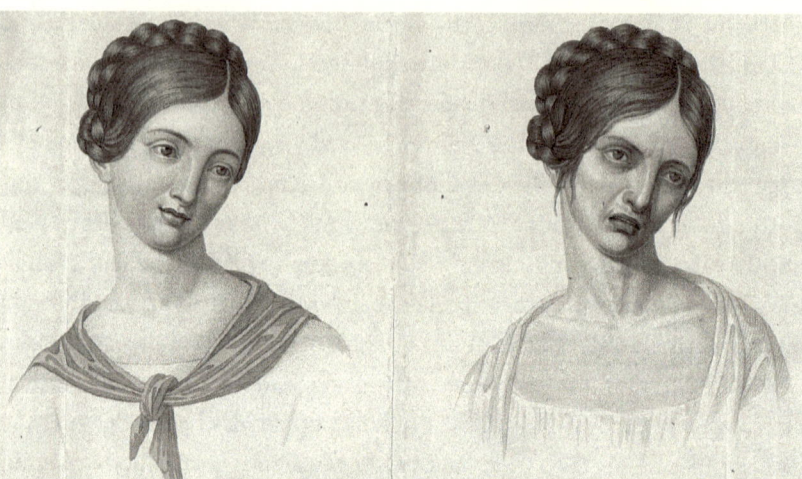

The ghastly face of cholera. A young woman who died of cholera, depicted when healthy and four hours before death. Colored stipple engraving, ca. 1831. (Wellcome Collection)

he would "blow out his brains at the first sign" rather than suffer through another bout.[49] One observer combined a graphic account of the symptoms to an even more graphic portrait of the victim's body: "The features changed like those of a corpse . . . coldness over the whole body . . . the most horrid martyrdom."[50] Even a patient clinging to life was described as "a living corpse."[51] The horrific, living-death like features of cholera's victims filled the press. Their skin "is deadly cold and shriveled, the voice nearly gone . . . the patient speaks in a whisper," wrote one.[52] People were "reduced to a shadow," "emaciated to a skeleton," wrote another.[53]

Perhaps the most graphic account published in an American paper came from a French hospital. An American visitor encountered a young woman convulsing with agony: "Her eyes were started from their sockets, her mouth foamed, and her face was of a frightful livid purple." It was indeed a "fiendish" and ghoulish sight, patients attempting to rise from their beds "like so many carousing corpses." Twenty or thirty death-like faces strained to catch the writer's eye as he sped through the ward, feeling "oppressed and half-smothered."[54]

Epidemic disease has always possessed the power to terrify. Yellow fever, in particular, could send communities into panic. It struck quickly, spread rapidly, and took a deadly, gruesome toll. Yet for all their faults, the physicians of 1793 confronting their health crisis always claimed some understanding of the threat. They could resort to graphic accounts of the disease. But these were most commonly offered within the construction of case histories, the morbid details compiled to facilitate diagnosis and treatment. The sort of gothic reaction common in 1832 was not voiced by physicians in 1793—but it was found in literature of the earlier period. Charles Brockden Brown lived through the yellow fever epidemic that swept New York in 1795, and he drew on this experience in writing two of his novels, *Arthur Mervyn* and *Ormond*. In both, his treatments anticipate the gothic portrayal of cholera in the 1830s; for that reason, a review of his narrative reveals just how far Americans' attitudes about disease had evolved, and their confidence in the ability of human senses to detect and unravel disease had diminished.

In *Arthur Mervyn,* serialized and published between 1798 and 1800, Philadelphia's yellow fever epidemic provides the backdrop for Brown's larger project. His literary objectives, as outlined in "Walstein's School of History. From the German Krants of Gotha," was to explore the behavior of good people coping with extraordinary stress. Brown and his circle believed that individuals could shape human society through "intellectual vigor," and that literature could serve society by "exhibiting a virtuous being in opposite conditions," thereby "displaying a model of right conduct."[55]

Brown's literary objectives aside, many have found in *Arthur Mervyn* a useful portrait of a city wrestling with yellow fever—a portrait that squares with nonfictional accounts of the epidemic. Mervyn, the protagonist, arrives to a diseased city all but deserted. The few people he meets on the street stink of the vinegar with which they have doused their clothes. Looters are everywhere; death carts hunt for the dead and dying left behind by their relatives. Similarly to the novel, journalist Mathew Carey, writing in the immediate aftermath of the 1793 Philadelphia epidemic, had lamented the "total dissolution of the bonds of society and dearest connections." Parents had abandoned their children, spouses their mates.

Even the recently orphaned children, now believed to be disease carriers, were shunned. According to reporter Carey and novelist Brown, this was a public no longer animated or restrained by the norms of civilized society.[56]

Brown also provides readers with a glimpse of the etiological debate. After speaking with a local doctor, Mervyn admits that his own contagionist ideas were naive and concedes that the disease must originate in local miasma. Brown's position is understandable—he was a close friend of Elihu Smith, Rush's student and the founder of the *Medical Repository*, which labored to canonize miasmatic theories of disease. But the darker, gothic qualities of the narrative were Brown's own. Whereas Smith would advance a position as optimistic as Rush's in reducing the fever to a treatable and ultimately manageable disease, Brown indulged in a gothic portrait that is less reassuring. Moreover, he embedded this within a larger statement about human nature—what we know and can know—that was far closer to the pessimism of the 1830s.[57]

Throughout the novel Mervyn finds himself lost within a confusing, unreadable maze of uncanny encounters and coincidences. Characters enter, disappear, and reenter his narrative in an almost farcical manner. The man who launches his urban adventure with a prank ends up being the person he unknowingly sets off to rescue from the plague. The villain who had years earlier seduced his sister bizarrely reappears as the caregiver of his duplicitous employer. Mervyn's universe is freakishly wired, yet he is hopelessly inept at interpreting and navigating it. He constantly misreads signs and charts misguided paths; even well-intentioned decisions have disastrous consequences. When he sets off heroically to save the fiancé of a character named Susan Hadwin, trapped in the disease-filled city, he decides to not reveal to other family members his purpose. Logical enough, but unaware of Mervyns's efforts, Susan's father sets off on the same errand to the infected city and as a result falls sick and dies. Moreover, the man Mervyn unselfishly saves for the sake of Susan absconds without returning to his betrothed, triggering a series of confusing events that lead to her death.

In failing to allow his protagonist to properly read his world and stitch together the chaotic events he encounters, Brown constructed a somewhat uncommon disease narrative. Within more conventional literary works, the disorder introduced into the characters'—and the readers'—lives by the arrival of disease is ultimately reconstituted by the author. That is, the unsettling experience of illness is ultimately cured and order is restored. But in *Arthur Mervyn,* this never occurs. Brown refused to reconnect all the pieces within a satisfying whole, denying his protagonist the ability to discover any sort of logic within the series of events and characters he encounters. And in doing so, Brown left us with a sense of what it means to live with—and remain under the disorder—of disease.[58]

In leaving his protagonist and his readers adrift, Brown constructed a narrative at odds with the literary conventions of his contemporaries. Instead, in his portrait of a dangerous city filled with malicious, predatory characters who feed on the naïveté of the innocent country boy, he told a story more in line with gothic conventions of a later era—and wholly out of sync with his contemporaries' sensibilities. Writing in the *North American Review,* William H. Gardiner complained that while Brown's novels were placed in America, his characters—"those dark monsters of the imagination"—bore no resemblance to any Americans Gardiner knew.[59] By 1832, however, Brown's portrait was far less out of step. As cholera jumped the Atlantic and crept south from Canada, many Americans came to believe that the world was filled with unpredictable dangers, and even worse, that human powers of perception and analysis were not up to the task of reading and decoding the world around them. In other words, Brown's hopelessly confused protagonist shared more with members of the Philadelphia cholera commission than Brown's contemporary Rush or good friend Smith.

Miasmatic theories of disease survived the cholera epidemic, but for many, critical underlying beliefs did not. Now many physicians retreated from the untempered confidence in science that had driven Rush and his friends while many laypeople lost faith in the power of their own senses to detect and read the threats to their persons. While the evidence of disease might still show on one's body—the red rash, the sallow complexion, the foul-smelling sore—the invading forces that threatened the body could no longer be so readily identified. There was no longer a stinking mound of rotting coffee at the end of Ball's Wharf to blame. Instead, disease drifted on the wind and welled from the earth, possessed the power to silently and invisibly cross mountains and oceans, following no predictable patterns and respecting no known laws. Nor, according to medical professionals, was our ability to decipher all this likely to change. The full significance of this for the prestige and credibility of American physicians—as well as Americans' own sense of their medical fates—was revealed a few years later during a series of puerperal fever epidemics.

The risks attached to childbirth were far from new in 1840. Nor were the symptoms of the deadly fever that often followed delivery unfamiliar. Virtually every doctor and midwife had encountered the elevated pulse, the distended belly, the alternating fever and chills, and the harsh odor that could appear within a just a few days of delivery—and the anguish that accompanied death.[60]

Explanations dated back millennia. Most, following the path laid out in the Hippocratic text *De mulierum morbis,* traced the illness to some sort of blockage or constriction that prevented the normal and necessary drainage of lochia or uterine fluid, leading to its accumulation and festering. A variation on this theory suggested that a mother's milk, which was widely believed to be menstrual fluid delivered through a duct from the uterus to the breast, could be blocked by anything from a swollen uterus to overly tight clothing, leading to the gathering of fetid matter in the womb. But most commonly, physicians believed that lochia that was not adequately discharged after birth remained in the new mother's body causing inflammation and fever. This festering material, possibly contained by the swollen uterus or constricted intestines, might be joined by similarly uneliminated fecal material, compounding the putrid toxins in the traumatized and thus vulnerable womb.[61]

Yet while explanations were ancient, the frequency and clustering of cases in the 1840s led physicians and expectant mothers to look more deeply at the disease. In 1842 there were twenty-nine fatal cases in one Vermont county and another twenty in Bath, New Hampshire. Similar clusters occurred in 1843 and 1844 in Ohio and New York. This was not a uniquely American phenomenon. In fact, European lying-in hospitals confronted mortality statistics even more shocking.[62]

On both continents, these clusters led some to suspect that the attending midwife or physician was in some way responsible. Oliver Wendell Holmes, the soon to be named professor of anatomy and physiology at Harvard, was far from the first to reach this conclusion. Almost fifty years earlier in 1795, Alexander Gordon of Aberdeen had concluded that physicians and midwives were conveying the contagion. He himself, he sadly admitted, was "the means of carrying the infection to a great number of women." But in America, Holmes was the most prominent and unequivocal in pointing the finger at his colleagues.[63]

After taking his M.D. at Harvard, Holmes had traveled to France where he studied under Pierre Charles Alexander Louis. Louis taught his students that most current medical therapies were useless and urged instead the aggregation of clinical data on which to base diagnoses and therapies. Inspired by this "numerical method," Holmes collected data on childbed fever and concluded that the doctor was the courier of the disease from patient to patient. While he could not identify the precise toxin or infecting agent, he was certain that childbed fever followed in the wake of only certain physicians—those who failed to take necessary precautions, like washing their hands and clothes, or waiting at least a day between attending a sick patient and delivering a child. The evidence was overwhelming, Holmes said. Doctors could no longer claim ignorance. And, therefore, fatal cases of childbed fever should be viewed as a "private pestilence . . . not as a misfortune but as a crime."[64]

Not everyone in the American medical community accepted Holmes's analysis. Charles Meigs, professor of obstetrics at Jefferson Medical College, denounced Holmes's condemnation of common birthing practices as the dark musings of the "weak minded." He conceded that the disease did seem to plague some practitioners more than others, but he attributed this to "strange, inexplicable coincidences." He answered Holmes's graphic accounts with his own story of a colleague who, after losing several patients to puerperal fever, left town for several days, shaved his head, and bought a new wig and new clothes before seeing his next laboring mother. But despite all these precautions—the sort advised by Holmes—his next patient contracted childbed fever and died. The doctor was not the source of the disease, concluded Meigs, and he was neither irresponsible nor criminal, "only unlucky."[65]

Perhaps recognizing the inadequacy of relying on coincidence and ill luck to explain the clustering of cases, Meigs offered his own scientific analysis. Following delivery, women were in an unusually weakened state. With their abdomens distended; suffering from new, open wounds; and with various cavities filled with "putrid juices," they were particularly vulnerable to some sort of threatening miasma. He could be no more specific than that in identifying the toxin that preyed on their weakened bodies. Perhaps it was some sort of "telluric poison," a foul emanation from the bowels of the earth that vitiated the air. But he could not really say: "No man hath known or can know what a miasm or a contagion is." The only good news was that this must be a relatively weak miasma, as it did not infect the attending practitioner or other family members, only the new mother, and as the disease was not universal, possibly only the weakest among them.[66]

Holmes's accusations and Meigs's weak response spoke to the disastrous state into which the profession had fallen, the no-win choice left to physicians in trying to explain an epidemic—either resort to ancient ideas about inexplicable miasmas or blame themselves, either ignore all the evidence of clustered occurrences or accept that for centuries they had been the vectors transporting fatal toxins from patient to patient. And concomitantly, the debate between Meigs and Holmes captured the horrible options left to patients trying to understand and treat the sicknesses that plagued them: either accept that their health was under constant attack by telluric poisons and earthly emanations, that a cluster of cases did not offer diagnostic clues, only evidence of bad luck, or the alternate explanation that their doctors, the practitioners they had turned to were often their worst enemy, that far from bringing science and the healing knowledge gathered through study and experience, they brought death.

7

Other Voices

PHARMACISTS, THOMSONIANS, AND HOMEOPATHS

While the majority of American physicians continued to embrace ancient theories of disease, there was some variety within the medical landscape during this period. As a result, Americans willing to look outside conventional practice for answers to their medical needs could find considerable innovation—alternative ideas, experimental movements—as well as a host of "irregular" practitioners who challenged not only conventional therapeutics but also the pessimism implicit within regular physicians' sober sense of medicine's potential. Many of these irregular practitioners were driven by their frustration with the sterility in conventional practice, but in developing their alternative pathway to good health, they recognized the need to address and incorporate the needs and beliefs of the lay public. In fact, as conventional practitioners strived to assert their authority over all things medical, these "other voices" actually made concessions to popular demands and constructed distributional infrastructures and diagnostic and research processes designed to make laypeople integral participants in their own medical care.

In this way, many of these movements left important marks on American medicine. But it is important not to overstate their actual impact on American disease theory—or even the extent to which they mounted a coherent etiological or therapeutic challenge to mainstream medical thought. In fact, in taking a brief look at a few of the challengers to "regular" physicians and their hegemony over the medical marketplace, it is important to sort out where their challenge actually lay: where they disagreed and ultimately agreed with the medical establishment they challenged.

For starters, it is worth noting that one prominent American journal was conspicuous in its relative silence on most things medical. Benjamin Silliman's *American Journal of Science,* launched in 1818, offered very little on the contentious questions surrounding disease, in particular its origins and transmissibility. In its first two decades—through the cholera epidemic of the 1830s—the journal did publish a couple of articles on fever and disease. Southwood Smith of the London Fever Hospital argued that malaria was caused by poison emanating from animal or vegetable substances. Echoing conventional miasmatic theory, he concluded that "certain stages of decomposition send forth miasmatic effluvia destructive to life." Another contributor delivered a more extensive article on malaria in 1830 in which they tied the disease to the poisonous exhalations peculiar to marshy areas. This analysis was also fairly conventional, fully in sync with most miasmatic theories. The author suggested that the toxic effluvia was "created by the joint action of heat and moisture, aided perhaps by electricity . . . upon decaying vegetables." The most intriguing hypothesis within the piece offered support for the widespread belief that frontier settlers were most susceptible to malaria. When the virgin forest floor was broken by plow, the writer argued, vegetable remains were exposed to heat and moisture, acquiring their toxic character. Inversely, once a cultivated region was abandoned, the soil began to build up another supply of vegetable matter waiting to be exhumed and converted to putrefaction. Turning on their head ideas about the healthful conditions of the frontier, this author argued that "pestilence walks in the footsteps of receding industry."[1]

The most direct engagement with the cholera epidemic was penned by William Henry, another English chemist. During the 1820s he had explored the ability of heat to disinfect certain commercial goods. Prompted by cotton importers worried about trade restrictions imposed in the wake of plague outbreaks, Henry tested the ability of intense heat to destroy the toxins within cotton yarn without impairing its character or quality.

Now, the spread of cholera encouraged Henry to renew his research on the disinfecting power of heat, ultimately concluding that temperatures above 140° rendered cowpox lymph inert but did not alter the character of yarn. More work was to be done—he envisioned a next set of experiments involving scarlatina, or scarlet fever, a bacterial disease identifiable by a bright red rash—but he was optimistic that processes might be found to sanitize certain commodities and shield them from the quarantine laws which were "aggressive and inadequate."[2]

Silliman's *American Journal of Science* would prove the most enduring of the period's scientific publications—it remains America's longest continuously produced scientific journal. True, it was more eclectic and comprehensive than the more narrowly focused medical journals, yet Silliman claimed to be willing to explore scientific questions related to health and disease. In fact, the statement of purpose in the premier issue promised to print articles on "comparative anatomy and physiology, and generally such other branches of medicine as depend on scientific principles." Nonetheless, between 1818 and 1835 the journal published very little on the most fundamental etiological questions troubling medical science.[3]

But then this was Benjamin Silliman's journal, and he was and still is recognized for the "pragmatic cast of his mind." A popular lecturer on the lyceum circuit and at the Lowell Institute, Yale's professor of "practical" chemistry, the founder of the New School of Applied Chemistry, and committed to "practical instruction in the applications of science to the arts and agriculture," it should not surprise us that he was uninterested in tiresome debates over the origins or contagiousness of major diseases—and seemingly indifferent, or perhaps even annoyed, by the ways in which chemistry was initially brought to bear in the search for an answer to yellow fever by men like Samuel Mitchill.[4]

Mitchill, Columbia's professor of chemistry and natural history, and Elihu Smith's collaborator and coeditor of the *Medical Repository*, offered a chemistry-based ancillary to Rush's miasmatic theories of disease that the *Repository* sought to enshrine. In *Remarks on the Gaseous Oxyd of Azote or of Nitrogene*, published in 1795, Mitchill argued that putrefaction generated the gaseous oxyd of azote, or "septon," which was the chemical agent of disease. His research further suggested that septon was largely an urban substance, produced in low-lying, waterside neighborhoods or poorly ventilated alleyways—and it was most abundant during warmer months. In other words, it was most prevalent in those areas and at those times where yellow fever was most commonly found, those areas in which the putrefying materials miasmatic theories blamed were most abundant.[5]

Several contributors to the *Medical Repository* echoed Mitchill's conclusions. Samuel Brown traced Boston's "pestilential disease" to the usual sources of putrefaction—rotting fish, spoiling beef, stagnant ponds—and the septon these produced, which he called "the matter and cause of all malignant or pestilential diseases." A Dr. Coit suggested that rotting fish was the primary source of the septic gas in New London, Connecticut. Henry Channing added overflowing privies to the list of suspects found in the same city, but the same chemical agent: septic gas.[6]

These fellow travelers seemed excited by the prospect of buttressing miasmatic theories with the authority accumulating in this emerging scientific field. And Mitchill himself offered up his conclusions as an example of the game-changing potential within chemistry made possible by the work of Antoine-Laurent Lavoisier. The French chemist had introduced new standards of investigatory rigor, a new model for laboratory research, as well as new understanding of respiration and combustion. But Mitchill's homage to Lavoisier aside, the American never brought to his studies the investigative rigor or commitment to empiricism of the French pioneer. Instead, his approach to the field was, according to one historian, more reliant on "logical deductions [and] imaginative leaps," his research less systematic than "fanciful and reverential—more contemplation of a kind of chemical sublime."[7]

In other words, Mitchill's approach to chemistry had much in common with the heroic ambitions of Benjamin Rush, more in common with his grand pursuit of huge answers than the empirically restrained Lavoisier or the pragmatically oriented Silliman. It is not surprising, therefore, that Silliman's journal avoided the etiological speculation of others, limiting itself to more narrowly argued pieces on chemistry and its practical applications to pharmacy. Wedged among submissions on physics, botany, and math, Silliman included entries on a variety of issues from "the respiration of oxygen gas in the affection of the thorax" to "a new process for Nitrous Ether." A Dr. Oliver submitted some thoughts on the "medical use" of Prussic acid; Dr. Miller provided a brief explanation of the use of Phosphoric acid on jaundice.[8] There were also multiple articles on pharmaceuticals. George W. Carpenter submitted most of these. He wrote lengthy reviews of Cinchona bark, opium, cantharides, and other drugs, describing their uses and the relative merits of different sources or preparations. And nestled within these reviews, he included a pitch for his own Carpenter's Saratoga Powders, derived from the healing waters of the famous hot springs.[9]

The difference in coverage—the relative neglect of fields within medical science other than chemistry and pharmaceuticals, the failure to engage in the larger questions surrounding disease origins and transmissibility—was seemingly explained in a contribution to Silliman's journal by George Wood, professor of materia medica and pharmacy at the newly established Philadelphia College of Pharmacy. In celebrating the opening of the college, he emphasized the increasing centrality of chemistry to medical science. While many physicians adhered mindlessly to a collection of ideas dating back to Galen, chemistry marched forward. In fact, Wood continued, the factor separating good from bad physicians, the factor separating advanced from archaic medical men, was their familiarity with chemistry.[10]

Philadelphia's new pharmacy school provided an institutional symbol of this linking of chemistry, pharmacy, and medical progress. In an 1833 contribution to the *American Journal of Science*, Wood stressed that pharmacy was a science, not a craft—the apothecary's work had moved beyond "the mere act of arranging and preparing" simple ingredients. And pharmacists were entitled to the status and authority commensurate with the scientific nature of their work. The new college also spoke to pharmacists' interest in professional autonomy. The University of Pennsylvania had established a masters of pharmacy degree in 1821, a year before the independent College of Pharmacy received its charter. But apothecaries resisted the university's attempt to place their profession under the auspices of the college and, by extension, the medical school. The only way that pharmacists could place their business "on a more respectable footing . . . as a branch of the science of medicine," they explained in their founding announcement, was through the "interposition and active agency of the druggists and apothecaries themselves."[11]

To further the new college's professional ambitions the founders quickly established a journal—the *Journal of the Philadelphia College of Pharmacy*. And Daniel Smith, the school's first president and journal's first editor, summarized the objectives of both institutions in his 1829 address to recent graduates. American pharmacy lagged dangerously behind European standards, he argued. There was virtually no statutory control, and most apothecaries had little scientific training. In fact, in too many towns, apothecaries, even those with training, were not adequately separated from the "wholesale druggist and the dealer in paints and dye stuffs" that had come to dominate the medical marketplace since the Revolution. The founders of the college had recognized these deficiencies—even their own, having been trained in the old way, "loosely and clumsily." But the new college would address these shortcomings, perhaps by adopting the French model. There, apothecaries served eight-year apprenticeships or a six-year apprenticeship combined with three courses of lectures. These were followed by extensive and rigorous public examinations.[12]

Much to pharmacists' annoyance, physicians were equally ready to point out the deficiencies within the pharmacy profession. A contributor to the *American Journal of Science* declared no profession "more liable to abuse" or so compromised by "ignorance and negligence." And this refusal to see pharmacists as anything close to equal partners in the medical profession was underscored during the physician-led efforts to construct a national pharmacopeia.[13]

The Philadelphia College of Physicians had first called for a comprehensive catalog of approved medicines and therapies in 1788. This project, like most early efforts of the college, quickly stalled. But in the second decade of the nineteenth century Samuel Mitchill and Lyman Spaulding led a renewed effort, leading to an 1820 Washington, D.C., conference called for the purpose of drafting a catalog of accepted pharmaceutical remedies. From the start, this project reflected the hierarchical sense of the medical community much earlier advanced by John Morgan in which physicians presided over surgeons and apothecaries within a three-tiered community. As the Massachusetts Medical Society stressed in 1808, "As it is the business of the physician to prescribe, and of the apothecary to prepare medicines," it was the exclusive responsibility of "the physicians as a body . . . to point out those articles of medicine, which they shall normally employ." Accordingly, when the National Medical Convention convened in January 1820, no pharmacists were invited. Organizers, intent that this be a truly "national" project, were pleased that there were physician delegates from Delaware, Connecticut, Maryland, Georgia, New York, Washington, and Pennsylvania—but their commitment to inclusion found no room for the apothecaries who would compound the medicines they canonized.[14]

The snub must have stung. Yet while excluded from this conference, pharmacists did find a satisfying opportunity in 1831 to weigh in when the *Journal of the Philadelphia College of Pharmacy* reviewed the second edition of *The Pharmacopeia of the United States of America,* which the Washington conference had first produced in 1820 and then revised in 1828. The first edition had been "marked throughout with the carelessness and undue haste of its preparations." But this newest iteration—drafted and published by a group of physicians in New York—was even worse. The reviewer filled more than twenty pages with examples of misnamed plants and medicines, inappropriate nomenclature, and incomplete descriptions. To the extent that these eminent physicians had sought to correct the shortcomings of the original edition, the author concluded, they had "utterly failed in their undertaking."[15]

The pharmacy journal was far from alone in trashing these editions of the pharmacopeia. Other journals were just as critical.[16] Still it is easy to see within this blistering critique the resentment pharmacists must have felt in being deemed irrelevant to this national project. And this was made even more clear when the same reviewer examined a different revision of *The Pharmacopeia of the United States* the following month. While one group of physicians had worked on revising the catalog in New York, an entirely separate group met in Washington in 1830 to prepare their own revision. Several drafts later, a committee drawn from the Washington group met in Philadelphia to finish their work. When they were done, they submitted the draft to a committee at the College of Pharmacy for its input. Once this revised edition—containing many "valuable practical" suggestions from the pharmacists—was published, the pharmacy journal was more positive—and appreciative—in its response. It was, in fact, with "honest pride and satisfaction" that the pharmacy college and journal celebrated this improved, and more inclusively constructed, pharmacopeia.[17]

While pharmacists were pleased that their efforts to elevate their professional status had been acknowledged by at least one group of physicians, it would be a mistake to reduce their objectives to finding common ground with physicians or to establishing some sort of collegial partnership in the marketplace. Their objectives were more complex. As an example, their strategy for dealing with the challenges represented by irregular practitioners and patent medicines was very different.

Daniel Smith had alluded to these challenges in his 1829 address in describing the troubling "encouragement given by our druggists to ignorant, idle, and drunken collectors of herbs and roots." Speaking to pharmacy college graduates in 1831, college vice president Henry Troth echoed this concern. The proliferation of bogus medicines and their "puffing" in the newspapers posed a threat to public health. But Troth was also quick to separate his position—and that of apothecaries more generally—from narrow-minded physicians who automatically denounced all medicines not dating back centuries. Some of the medicines they rejected as outside the medicinal canon were actually "valuable."[18]

It was an interesting position—one that separated pharmacists from most regular physicians, and one that further staked out pharmacists' distinctive place within the medical community. Troth served notice that pharmacists would sit at the scientific cutting edge of medical care, not mindlessly attached to tired old therapeutics but instead serving as arbiters of the useful and scientific among the host of irregular therapies and drugs entering the medical marketplace. And to demonstrate this distinctive position, the pharmacy college decided as one of its first major initiatives to ascertain and then publish the "most appropriate" formulas for eight leading patent medicines. Rather than simply denounce, like the regular-physician establishment, the patent medicines that filled American pantries, the college would provide consumers and apothecaries the tools to properly evaluate them.

Dozens of British patent medicines had entered the American market in the previous century. Rendered "scientific" by their complex formulas and distinctive by their readily identifiable bottles, these medicines were distributed by all sorts of shopkeepers—tailors, booksellers, grocers, post offices—as well as apothecaries. Their supply was interrupted by the imperial conflict, but American consumers were not to be denied, and so American producers began to imitate or approximate their formulas as well as their packaging. In the first decades of the nineteenth century more and more American entrepreneurs entered this market, inspiring spinoff industries such as bottle-making to supply the distinctive glass containers.[19]

But while these American knockoffs might look the same, there were vast differences in their actual contents. The College of Pharmacy committee tasked with identifying the "actual" formula for the leading medicines found that one recipe for Bateman's Pectoral Drops distributed in the United States called for a 1/1000 ratio of opium to other liquid ingredients. In another (perhaps more popular) iteration, the ratio was 1/14.[20]

The committee completed its work in 1824. Extracting from the multiple recipes for each medicine the ingredients they deemed most useful, and adding new ingredients they believed would strengthen the medicine's original therapeutic purpose, they published a list of standardized formulas along with the recommendation that future packaging be stripped of all "extravagant pretensions and false assertions." The formulas, reprinted in 1833 and 1839, provided apothecaries and drug manufacturers with an invaluable tool. But pharmacy as a profession was actually the greatest beneficiary. This project advanced pharmacists' position as the scientifically trained arbiters of pharmaceutical therapy within the marketplace without alienating vast portions of the public that believed in and relied on these patent medicines.

In their sensitivity to this public demand, pharmacists were more realistic than physicians. The explosion of the patent (or more typically proprietary) medicine industry over the first half of the century meant that American consumers could choose from a host of tonics to rouse themselves from lethargy and several blood purifiers to remove the toxins that impeded delivery of nutrients to their tired bodies. They could cleanse their gut through an assortment of cathartics and boost their blood's oxygen content with one of many oxygenators. By midcentury, leading manufacturers like the Ayer Company had stumbled on the idea of promoting their products through the publication of annual almanacs. But earlier—and perhaps even more effectively—these companies hawked their goods in the rapidly expanding network of newspapers, whose dependence on advertising revenues was greater than their commitment to marketing veracity.[21]

Pharmacists clearly recognized that the public's demand for patent medicines could not be ignored. Any hopes to advance their profession—and secure their livelihoods—depended on accepting this commercial reality. But in doing so they were as much cagey as realistic. For in adopting this stance they assumed a place in the medical field separate from physicians in terms of expertise and therapeutic approach. Moreover, in choosing to not reject all of these medicines and therapies as mere quackery, the committee identified pharmacists as the scientific arbiters of quality drugs. It was a position that staked out their professional turf while advancing their practical interests. As the committee concluded, this project elevated their reputation while "extending the drug business of our city."[22]

It was an ingenious but somewhat risky strategy as it placed pharmacists on something of a tightrope, simultaneously staking their professional credibility on their scientific training, especially in the field of chemistry, while also tolerating or even implicitly approving certain medicines of more questionable origins. It was a strategy that might ingratiate themselves with the patent medicine–buying public but one that put them in bed with the commercial drug industry and left them vulnerable to allegations that they were complicit in the advance of unscientific, or at best "irregular," practices.

Among the "irregular" challenges to pharmacists and physicians in the first quarter of the nineteenth century, the most significant came from Samuel Thomson. To a public desperate for a theory of disease and a therapeutic program offering greater hope—or at least the pretense of greater certainty—his populist challenge to the medical establishment was well timed. For pharmacists, Thomson's botanical-based therapeutics offered a test of their ability to establish control over, while neither condemning nor even distancing themselves from, Americans' drug-taking habits.

Born in 1769, Samuel Thomson was raised on a farm in Alstead, New Hampshire. His father was a harsh taskmaster, and Samuel grew to hate the work, along with the stern doctrines of his father's Baptist faith. Samuel did, however, take an interest as a child in botanical and herbal remedies. The "Widow Benton" introduced him to the powers of local herbs, including lobelia, which would anchor the medical system that made him famous.[23]

But Thomson's medical philosophy, as relayed in his autobiography, was driven as much by his contempt for conventional medicine as his interest in local plants and herbs. After severely cutting his ankle in 1788, the poultice advised by a local physician exacerbated the injury, leading Thomson to devise his own cure: a combination of comfrey root and turpentine. Two years later, after his mother was struck down by galloping consumption, Thomson refused the doctor's prescription after he also fell ill and subsequently survived. His most significant lesson in the futility of conventional medicine was learned after his wife fell seriously ill after giving birth to their first child. Thomson summoned six doctors who all pursued some combination of bleeding and purging, only to see her condition deteriorate. At that point, he summoned a local root doctor under whose care his wife fell senseless for three days, broken only by spasms "so violent they jarred the whole house." After that she was "raving distracted" for three days, then "perfectly stupid" for three days. She then laughed for three days and then cried for three more. But after this biblical ordeal, she recovered. She was never again quite right, Thomson acknowledged, and the whole episode, he complained, set him back more than two hundred dollars. But he was fully converted to the power of herbal medicine and immediately apprenticed with the miracle-working root doctor.[24]

For the next few years Thomson limited his practice to members of his own family. He successfully removed the canker from his two-year-old daughter's eye, although the "sight came out with it." And he cured his son's croup with rattlesnake oil. With his reputation as a healer growing, he decided in 1805 to abandon farming and offer his services as a physician. First, however, he felt he must systematize his methods; if he was to pursue this as a business, he must "fix upon some system . . . that might be easily taught to others."[25]

Thomson's brilliance lay in developing a simple, intuitively logical theory of health and disease that allowed common people to both assess and treat their ailments. It was not all that unconventional. In fact, he grounded his system in a simplified version of humoral theory: The body was composed of four elements; poor health was due to a systemic failure (most commonly tied to poor digestion), which left the body unable to generate the heat needed for good health. Nor were Thomson's therapeutics that far removed from those of regular physicians who tried to restore health through various methods of regulating the body's secretions. But Thomson abandoned the conventional methods of bleeding and sweating for a simple course of herb-based drugs.[26]

As the goal was to raise the body's temperature, Thomson started his patients off with "Medicine #1," or lobelia, an herbal purgative prescribed to quickly but only temporarily raise internal temperature. This was followed by "Medicine #2," most typically capsicum, sometimes laced with black pepper and ginger, and designed to sustain for a longer period the heat elevated by Medicine #1. The remaining medicines that made up his pharmacy added nuances to the treatment. Medicine #3 would scour the stomach and remove cankers; Medicine #5, a syrup consisting of plant derivatives that functioned as tonics, such as bayberry root, mixed with sugar and brandy, were intended to stimulate the body toward balance and health.[27]

It is not hard to imagine the attraction of a system that did not break too far from conventional medical science but also appealed to the demands for self-treatment growing within the medical marketplace since the eighteenth century. Thomson's ideas were easy to grasp, his therapies were easy to use, and the instructions and rights to its use were affordable. Moreover, Thomson distributed his system through a pyramid-type network that invited believers to share in the profits while crossing state and regional lines. Over the next two decades his agents sold more than 100,000 patents and his book went through thirteen editions. Customers purchased their medicines through licensed stores and supply depots that competed directly with regular pharmacists. Thomson claimed that by the 1830s his methods were being employed by more than 3 million people. Contemporaries estimated that ten thousand Bostonians and half of the residents of Ohio were Thomsonians. Mississippi's governor calculated that half of all Mississippians followed the botanical regimen.[28]

Thomson and the medical movement he inspired reflected larger currents within Jacksonian America. His attack on regular physicians resonated with the anti-intellectualism manifested in everything from Second Great Awakening evangelicalism to legal codifiers' attacks on the common law.[29] While Thomson did not reject the value of education altogether, he did mock the counterintuitive methods that established medical schools taught, and he suggested that no amount of education would make a fool wise or a doctor lacking the "natural gift" an effective healer. The forty Thomsonian journals published during the movement's heyday were reflective of the antebellum expansion of print culture. And with his licensing and distribution schemes, Thomson skillfully tapped into the entrepreneurial culture exploding in conjunction with America's expanding commercial infrastructure.[30]

The overlapping between Thomsonianism and the religious innovation of the period is particularly striking. Thomson suggested that he was bringing to medicine the same sort of democratic transparency earlier brought to religion through the Protestant Reformation and government through the American Revolution. The embrace of his system by not only mainstream evangelicals but also those on the fringes of the Second Great Awakening—Latter-day Saints and Shakers—suggest that he was not entirely mistaken in his sense of his work. His agents blanketed the nation much like the Methodist circuit riders of earlier revivals, and many of his licensed distributors were Shakers. It is more than coincidence that when Thomson decided to bring better order to his growing distribution network, he hired Elias Smith, a former itinerant preacher and leader of the unorthodox evangelical movement known as the Christian Connection.[31]

But while Thomsonianism found sympathetic currents within many aspects of Jacksonian America, it was the failure of conventional medicine that opened most wide the door to this movement. The methods and practices of regular physicians were simply too vulnerable to criticism. How logical was bleeding, Thomson asked, when everyone knows that excessive blood loss leads to death? Why apply a blister, in effect a second wound, to cure a first? And how could regular physicians defend their "exorbitant" fees when they could guarantee so little?[32]

Thomson filled his autobiography with story after story of patients whom conventional medicine had failed: a three-hundred-pound woman tortured by convulsive fits, another with a tumor on her breast the size of an egg. Many of his patients suffered from long-term illnesses and were now willing to try almost anything to secure relief: a parent whose son was afflicted with a fever sore for seven years, a woman who had been confined to her bed for over a decade and was now being cared for by her young adult children. Embedded within many of these accounts was a concomitant anger at the regular physicians who failed to heal but still charged their patients, such as the parents of a child unsuccessfully treated with mercury, who paid "twenty-five dollars for killing the child by inches."[33]

The severity of conventional therapeutics contributed to these frustrations. A man complained of his son's suffering after being treated for a chronically bleeding nose with a corrosive sublimate snuff. Another woman was exhausted after enduring forty-two bleedings in two years. But they did not turn to Thomson looking for a kinder and gentler course of treatment. Lobelia was no walk in the park. In fact, it was labeled "screw-agur" by Thomson's critics as well as "belly-my-grizzle" and "ram cat." Thomson liked to emphasize that it was a natural, herbal purgative rather than a mineral one like calomel. But there was no denying that his "pukeweed" was a harsh and demanding medicine.[34]

Yet it was not the severity of its therapeutics that broke the movement. Ultimately, Thomsonianism collapsed under its own weight. Thomson struggled in particular to control the expansive distribution network that he created. Agents, both licensed and rogue, negotiated their own prices and refused to honor reimbursement agreements earlier struck with Thomson. Unlicensed pharmacists pedaled his patented medicines without compensation. Even protégé Elias Smith published a *Medical*

Pocketbook that lifted Thomson's entire system and sold it for five dollars, a fourth the price of Thomson's original guide.[35]

Another former agent, Alva Curtis, mounted a challenge to Thomson of a more enduring kind. He sought to boost the profile and prestige of Thomsonian medicine through the establishment of botanical colleges and a professional association for practitioners. He launched the first of these colleges—the Botanico-Medical School of Columbus—in his own home in 1839, institutionalizing the division between him and Thomson, between those who shared his vision of a cadre of professional botanical practitioners and Thomson's more democratic true believers.

The popularity of Thomsonian medicine challenged both regular physicians and pharmacists. And the response of many was to simply incorporate botanical therapies into their practices. Just as a wing within the botanical movement drifted toward the center in search of greater acceptance and respectability, more and more members within the conventional medical community met them. Pharmacists in particular, always more agile than regular physicians in responding to this sort of threat, added more botanical therapies to their medicine cabinets—so many, in fact, that they made Thomsonian leaders furious. They claimed to be suspicious of pharmacists' sloppy practices, worried that their botanicals would be tainted with impure ingredients. But the real threat lay in the danger that pharmacists might coopt the movement and cut into the profits of Thomsonian depots and distributors.[36]

But while individual pharmacists and some regular physicians made concessions to the movement, at the institutional level, within the societies and organizations that represented the two professions, physicians and pharmacists maintained very different attitudes. Regular physicians, even while acknowledging the possibilities within some of Thomson's botanicals, mocked his broader theories and tried to criminalize Thomsonian practitioners through state licensing statutes. But when they failed—in fact, when their efforts only served to increase opposition to these statutes, leading to their repeal in the 1830s and 1840s—physicians rather than retreat adopted a more comprehensive strategy aimed at suppressing all medical "fads, quacks and cure-alls." Joined together within the newly formed American Medical Association (AMA), regular physicians passed resolution after resolution condemning irregular practices and medicines and campaigned to suppress their promotion.[37]

Collectively gathered within the AMA and other state medical associations, regular physicians maintained their hostility toward Thomsonian and other irregular practitioners through the century. Even during the Civil War, with northern military officials desperate to expand the Union Army medical corps, regular physicians succeeded in prohibiting irregular physicians from applying. Even though roughly half of all applicants boasting the approved medical school degrees failed to pass the army medical exam, the AMA and other organizations refused to alter their stance.[38]

There was more than a little hypocrisy in their high-minded position. Medical journals continued to advertise patent medicines throughout the nineteenth century. Yet still, the position of the AMA was very different from the more accommodating position laid out by Troth in 1831 and maintained fairly consistently by pharmacy leaders throughout the century. Not every pharmacist was comfortable with this sacrificing of the scientific high road, but the realists within the profession prevailed. For example, when the American Pharmaceutical Association (APA) formed in 1852, a first order of business was the adoption of a code of ethics that forbade any association with "secret formulas and the practice arising from a quackish spirit." But immediately members pointed out that many of them depended on the sale of patent medicines and irregular, even "quack" remedies to support their more scientific contributions. As a result, the APA made adherence to the code nonobligatory. Over the next several decades, the code all but disappeared from APA literature, leading the AMA to attack pharmacists for protecting patent medicines and unscientific therapies. Despite the AMA's opposition, pharmacists defended their conciliatory stance well into the twentieth century, arguing that these therapies were vital to both their practices and their customers who relied on them—and for them to do more than prohibit dangerous nostrums "would be to ask us to sacrifice the interests of the people for the selfish benefit of physicians."[39]

In this way, pharmacists did stake out a fairly consistent and distinctive strategy in dealing with Thomson and other irregular insurgents, including the patent medicines that remained so popular with the public. But if in doing so they preserved a place within the medical mainstream for Thomson's ideas, it is important to be careful about stating exactly what this movement did and did not represent. Thomsonianism demonstrated the extent of disaffection, at least among certain portions of the American public, with conventional medicine. It suggested an openness to alternative therapeutics, which seemed both simple and "natural" gifts of the world in which they lived. Thomsonianism tells us that the burgeoning democratic spirit of Jacksonian America touched multiple aspects of American culture. And that innovators—or entrepreneurs—able to understand the needs of American patients—and consumers—would find accessible markets. But in terms of the movement's impact on American disease theory—on its fundamental contribution to the science of medicine—the movement offered little. Thomson built his system on ancient humoral theories, and while he and his followers rejected specific measures, they did not reject a therapeutic culture that assumed disease needed to be fought into submission—a culture that believed there was no easy path to good health. Just as Rush's followers seemed to embrace the harshness of his methods and correlate the demands of the treatment with the severity of the disease, Thomson recognized that cure lay in demanding rounds of purging and sweating.

And consequently, to the extent that pharmacists managed to corral this movement, chasten at least in part its more bizarre elements, and absorb some of the promise within its botanical alternatives, they did not do much to advance medical science.

There is another aspect of Thomsonian medicine worth emphasizing: It drew greatest support from the less affluent. Thomson's greatest influence was in the West. Of his 167 authorized agents in 1833, 41 worked in Ohio, 29 in Tennessee, 21 in Alabama, and 11 in Indiana. The bulk of his followers came from more modest parts of the public. Another movement to challenge the theories and therapeutics of conventional physicians and pharmacists—homeopathy—found its strength in a different class and different part of the country. More nuanced and complex in both its diagnostic and therapeutic prescriptions, homeopathy made its greatest gains in the urban Northeast among better-educated and more affluent folks apparently frustrated with conventional therapeutics. Even many practicing physicians embraced its ideas and incorporated them into their practices. And in doing so, they embraced a very different but ultimately no more modern belief about disease.[40]

Homeopathy was the contribution of a German physician named Samuel Hahnemann.[41] Brought to America by Hans Gram in 1828, Hahnemann's ideas slowly spread over the next decade before reaching widespread acceptance in the 1840s. Hahnemann stumbled on the central element of his medical theory while researching the effects of cinchona, a South American tree whose bark contains quinine. Studying this "Peruvian bark," which was widely recognized as an effective treatment for malaria, he applied the substance to himself and soon exhibited malaria-like symptoms even though he was perfectly healthy. The observation yielded the central principle of his medical theory: "To cure mildly, rapidly, certainly, and permanently, choose, in every case of disease, a medicine which can itself produce an affection similar to that sought to be cured." This "law of similars" (similia similibus curantur), commonly reduced to the maxim "like is cured by like," sent Hahnemann on a hunt for other substances that produced in healthy people a set of symptoms that paralleled those found in individuals suffering from particular diseases. Believing that what sickens the healthy cures the sick, he applied the same substance to the sick individual, theorizing that the symptoms and hence the underlying disease would be cured.[42]

Part of Hahnemann's appeal was that he invited other physicians and even nonprofessionals to join in the search for these medicinal substances. These "provings" must be systematic—careful records must be kept of dosage, the reaction of test subjects to a particular substance must be observed and meticulously recorded. Yet the appeal was general—and clearly attractive to laypeople with a rigorous curiosity in health and disease as well as professionals anxious to identify alternative treatments. The provings were subsequently published in homeopathic journals, with the ever-growing compilation of experiments providing a complex but navigable catalog for professionals and laypeople intrigued by the prospect of diagnosing and treating illness.[43]

The battery of provings also led homeopathy toward a second critical principle summed up in the law of minimum dose. As more and more experiments were conducted, the dosage recommended to achieve the cure decreased. Critics seized on this law, ridiculing the minuscule doses recommended to achieve a cure. Oliver Wendell Holmes, a Harvard-trained physician and future Parkman Professor of Anatomy and Physiology at the Harvard Medical School, pointed out that one drop of tincture of chamomile, diluted according to homeopathic prescription, would yield 5 billion doses for every person in the world, past and present. But Hahnemann argued that these critics failed to recognize the process by which the latent powers within a substance were excited or animated through the preparatory process. Practitioners were advised to mix the substance with water or alcohol so that the curative powers could be "potentized," thereby releasing medicinal powers far greater than the minuscule dosage would suggest.[44]

Some fans have credited homeopathy with leading the fight against the ancient therapeutic practices still dominating American medical practice. In the substitution of particularized, carefully modulated medicines they see a half-step toward modern drug regimens—medicines that were more carefully dosed and more specifically targeted toward specific ailments. And it is true that homeopathic practitioners did substitute ever-diminishing doses targeting specific symptoms for the gut-wrenching and depleting rigors of conventional medicine. But homeopathy was far from modern in its premises. For starters, the almost magical amplification of a substance's curative powers through "potentization" or "dynamization" revealed that Hahnemann's fundamental theory drew more from the mysticism of vitalism than the disciplines of biology or chemistry.

Moreover, in celebrating the power of these agents to inspire good health, homeopaths shared a critical premise with the heroic practitioners of the nineteenth century. While other reformers argued that practitioners should act with modesty, that drugs and other treatments should take a backseat to the healing powers of nature, that "modern medicine" should concentrate on pain management while gently assisting the body's intrinsic curative powers, homeopaths joined physicians like Benjamin Rush who scorned the timidity within this approach. Nature, Hahnemann argued, could be a useful asset in preserving the health of the healthy but could not cure disease. In fact, nature could respond to illness in dangerously counterproductive ways. When the vital forces key to the preservation of good health were subverted by some external force, the body's natural reaction was to fight back. But these defensive measures—evacuations, metastasis, the elimination of fluids—often constituted, in effect, a second illness. In other words, left to its own devices, the body was a danger to itself—only the intervention of a skilled practitioner could protect the body from self-harm.[45]

Hahnemann also moved in an even more markedly antimodern direction when he rejected the idea that discrete foreign entities were responsible for illness. Instead, he argued that this search for the causes of disease, this "materialist" approach that believed disease was caused by a substance or thing and that cure lay in removing this "imagined and presumed material cause of the disease," was a fantasy. Rather, disease was a "dynamic disarrangement of our spirit-like vital principle in sensations and function."[46]

In explaining his vitalist understanding of disease, Hahnemann suggested that physicians were fooled by the discharges accompanying disease. In the foul evacuations, the secretion of pus and sweat, they leapt to the erroneous conclusion that they were seeing the morbific material that was agent of the disease, whereas in truth these excretions were "nothing more than products of the disease." In this conclusion Hahnemann was essentially correct, but in denying all value in digging beneath these "products," he staked out a position contrary to the sort of thinking that would enable medicine to move beyond its etiological stagnation. Isaac Cathrall had conducted elaborate experiments in 1794 on the black matter associated with yellow fever—even rubbing it on his own lips and tongue to see if it was the agent or product of the disease. But homeopaths pursued no similar questions or experiments. They did not share the fundamental confidences of theoreticians like Rush or Cathrall that the cause of disease could be ascertained. Instead, the origins were beyond human comprehension and therefore impossible to unravel.[47]

In this sense homeopathy was more in tune with the diagnostic fatalism that replaced the theoretical ambitions of the late eighteenth century. While intellectually optimistic in their belief that lay and professional practitioners could treat illness through the compilation of a vast catalog of curative agents, homeopaths made no commitment to uncovering the origins of disease. At best they would approach it through the backdoor—treating the symptoms with the belief that in doing so they would cure the mysterious and never-knowable source of the disease itself.

The distance between homeopathy and the more scientific direction being taken by more modern medical visionaries was made clear when a group of reformers in Hahnemann's movement tried to establish a chair of pathology and diagnostics at the homeopathic school in Philadelphia. Their efforts led to a schism and the founding of a separate school, the Hahnemann Medical College. The laboratory at the new school symbolized the etiological gap between the two factions. Traditional homeopaths did not believe this sort of clinical research was necessary to diagnose illness or understand disease. Physicians were trained to develop a therapeutic regimen by conducting elaborate interviews, acquiring a detailed, personalized understanding of the symptoms to be pharmaceutically treated. There was little to be learned in the lab as the focus of the homeopath's efforts was the patient's particular symptoms, not the unknowable abnormality beneath. As Hahnemann urged his followers, "treat the patient, not the disease."[48]

Other health movements emerged during these years, offering varying degrees of logic and value. Sylvester Graham's advice regarding diet, sex, and hygiene provided a reasonable set of rules for healthy living that probably did more good than harm. Hydropathy similarly offered real health benefits—physiologically and psychologically—especially for women. But the theoretical content within these movements was thin. Neither offered a comprehensive theory of disease nor attempted to understand the root causes of illnesses. Neither represented any sort of significant departure from conventional health philosophy nor contributed to the actual science that would revolutionize medicine in the last decades of the century. In fact, the culmination of all the medical creativity of the era was the emergence of the eclectics, a movement committed to weaving together the most effective therapies drawn from a variety of movements. Drawing heavily from the botanical principles of Samuel Thomson and others like Wooster Beach and Samuel Rafinesque, but adamantly refusing to be hamstrung by any single system, the eclectics promoted a theory-empty medical chest of therapies devoid of any unifying or explanatory vision other than the commitment to curative efficacy.[49]

And although pharmacists should be recognized for adopting a more flexible approach to these alternative therapies, acknowledging the importance of chemistry to modern medicine, and working to elevate professional training and standards, through the middle of the century they could claim relatively few concrete therapeutic or professional gains. For example, while chemistry was taught at the Philadelphia College of Pharmacy from the beginning, during the first several decades this training was more technical than scientific. Pharmacy students would hear a series of chemistry lectures but there were no labs.[50] The college did not build its first chemistry lab until 1870 and its first microscopical lab until 1882.[51] And despite pharmacists' aspirations to represent the cutting edge of medical science, they moved no faster than physicians in embracing germ theory. While the *Journal of the Philadelphia College of Pharmacy* generally voiced support for the emerging science, articles advancing contrary disease theories—ones competing with the conclusions reached by Robert Koch and others—were published in the journal as late as 1885.[52]

Pharmacists did succeed in winning a seat at the table in the decennial revisions of the national pharmacopeia. In fact, in 1877 the management and revising of *The Pharmacopeia of the United States* was turned over entirely to pharmacists. But physicians still encroached on their turf and exercised authority over those who mixed their drugs. In several states, licensing statutes allowed physicians to compound drugs and granted to them the authority to examine prospective pharmacists. Pharmacists would not gain more complete control over their profession and establish occupational and intellectual autonomy until late in the century, when the advancing science forced specialization—when the sheer amount of medical knowledge being accumulated forced the parsing out of this scientific knowledge and therapeutic task. Probably the most telling indicator of eventual pharmacist autonomy is reflected in the fact that by 1900, pharmacy and materia medica had all but disappeared from medical school curricula.[53]

In other words, while noteworthy for their interest in helping medical science break free of the lethargy that plagued regular physicians, in practice they advanced the conversation very little. As a result, the most significant challenge to conventional theories of health and disease would not come from pharmacists or any of the irregular movements that added energy, if not substance, to the conversation. Instead, the most intriguing and promising challenge to established etiology and therapeutics would be launched by an individual who succeeded in gathering virtually no following for his medical ideas during his lifetime.

Josiah Nott entered the debate over yellow fever and disease more generally through a series of articles published in the 1840s and 1850s. While his animalcular theories were largely rejected in his own time, they are now viewed by some medical historians as the most promising avenue left unpursued during the decades before the revolutionary discoveries of Robert Koch. Nott's racial theories, on the other hand, drew to him a wide following in his time and contempt in ours. What is less recognized is that his medical and racial ideas were not disconnected. Instead, they should be viewed as products of a unified sense of the natural order—a sense of biology and history that allowed him to imagine etiological ideas that were commendable in their foresight alongside racial ideas that were damnable in their bigotry.

8

Voices Ignored

FROM ANTONIE VAN LEEUWENHOEK TO JOSIAH CLARK NOTT

IN SEPTEMBER 1853 JOSIAH Nott watched helplessly as yellow fever spread past the edges of Mobile, Alabama, toward the rural community of Spring Hill, where his family had taken refuge for the summer. Nott, the city's most prominent physician, was all too familiar with the disease—it had struck Mobile in 1837, 1839, 1842, and 1843. Mild outbreaks also occurred in 1844 and 1847, but as the death count rose in the last week of August 1853, Nott braced for a more serious visitation.[1]

The doctor had not taken complete comfort in sending his family to the country. The irregular pattern of earlier epidemics had convinced him that neither contagionist nor miasmatic theorists were correct in their explanation for the disease. In 1837 yellow fever had surfaced in a part of the city far removed from the docks, dispelling, it seemed, any suggestion that it had arrived via ship. In 1839 the disease first appeared in clean, well-ventilated neighborhoods, challenging those who argued that yellow fever welled from the putrefying filth of low-lying slums. Yet Nott was still unprepared for the tragedy that lay ahead. By mid-September the fever had reached the household of his in-laws at Spring Hill. Within a span of two weeks, four of his own children had been infected with the disease and died.[2]

Six months later Nott described—or perhaps more accurately reflected on—the disease that had taken his children. He had previously believed that the young were comparatively immune to yellow fever, yet in 1853 they had been "generally and violently attacked." Even more painfully, he questioned his previous confidence that the disease was not

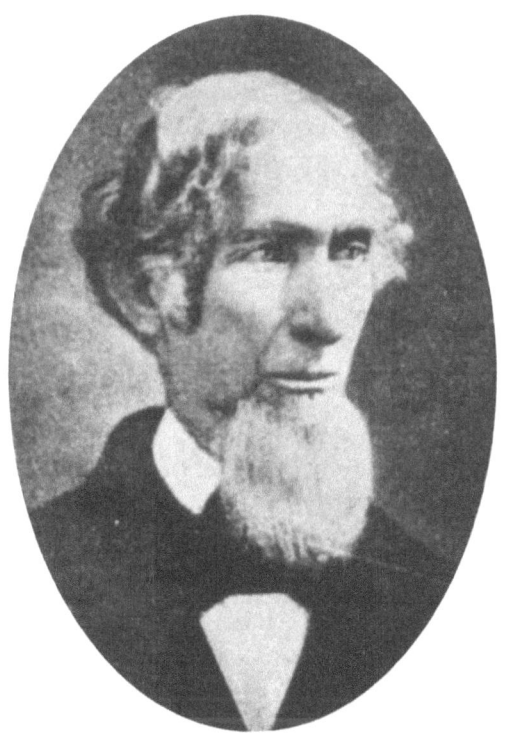

Josiah Nott, a prominent southern physician who broke with conventional thought in advancing animalcular theories of disease, n.d. (National Library of Medicine)

contagious, that it could not be communicated from person to person. While perhaps true in past epidemics, the events of the last year left him "leaning" toward the belief that one victim could through some means pass the disease on to another. Beneath this change of opinion—and separated within the text by six pages—Nott admitted that on 12 August he had attended a man, Alfred Murray, in Mobile suffering from yellow fever and had recommended that he be removed to a relative's home in Spring Hill. Within three weeks, two of Murray's host's children had been infected with the disease. In less than a week, yellow fever had struck the nearby home of James Deas, Nott's father-in-law. As Nott counted the number of deaths within Spring Hill over the next few weeks—five whites, two people of mixed-race, and one Black—he chose not to say that four of the five white people killed were his own children. Nor did he explicitly acknowledge what he must have privately feared: that their deaths were directly linked to the patient Nott sent into the previously disease-free community.³

Nott's brief account in the *New Orleans Medical and Surgical Journal* was as remarkable as it was tragic—in part in that he could offer a clinical review of the disease that had devasted his family just six months earlier, in part in that he would publicly acknowledge that certain critical elements of his medical understanding had been shaken, but most of all in that he would offer a thinly veiled admission of his own culpability. Yet within this painful *mea culpa,* one element of his understanding of yellow fever was unchanged. The events of 1853 had further convinced him that conventional theories regarding the disease were inadequate. The speed with which yellow fever reached into the hinterlands, the idiosyncratic way in which the disease leapfrogged houses and families, offered proof of the argument he had first advanced in 1848 that yellow fever was in some way connected to insects.

By midcentury yellow fever was primarily a southern disease. Northern officials linked their relative immunity to the preventative measures they had launched in the aftermath of earlier epidemics. In cities like Philadelphia, New York, and Boston, the ad-hoc committees formed during earlier crises all morphed into permanent public health committees focused primarily on cleaning up their environments. For example, in Philadelphia, where city officials had long operated under the belief that health and disease were linked to environmental conditions, the epidemics of the 1790s inspired increased dedication to cleaner urban conditions and more pure water. By the end of the decade, the city had adopted improved methods for cleaning streets and launched an ambitious plan to deliver pure water to city residents. In 1799 the city adopted Benjamin Latrobe's proposal that steam engines be utilized to draw water from the Schuylkill River into a settling tank at the city center before being pumped into an elevated reservoir. After passing through four epidemic years, city officials were willing to spend as much as a quarter million dollars on a network of pumps, reservoirs, and cast-iron mains and wooden distribution pipes.⁴

Acknowledging that public health required public cooperation, Philadelphia city officials also adopted measures to educate its citizens: health advice was published in the newspapers and distributed in pamphlets. Officials also monitored compliance by collecting information from physicians and even paid informers. They regularly inspected the jail, almshouse, and hospital. And in 1795, when yellow fever reappeared, they formed a citizens' committee to enforce sanitation measures and report violations.[5]

Philadelphia also took steps to establish a more effective system of maritime interception and quarantine. There was simply too much evidence that the earlier quarantine system anchored by an inspection station at State Island was too porous. It was a reasonable distance from the city—seven miles by water and five by land—and it housed a hospital where the suspected sick could be quartered until proven safe for entry. But the city's Board of Health identified too many holes in the system, too many ships, cargos, and passengers that avoided interception. And so, in 1801 they opened a new inspection station and "Lazaretto" on Tinicum Island.[6]

The new site was farther from the city (13 miles) and more thorough in its inspection processes and rigorous in their enforcement. Incoming ships were greeted by a quarantine official and physician and then inspected for any signs of disease or putrefaction. The ship's officers were interrogated about their voyage, the ports they had entered in enroute to Philadelphia, and the health of all those on board. And if either inspection or interrogation raised any suspicion, the ship would be detained while its cargo was offloaded and aired, its hold fumigated, and its crew carefully observed for any signs of disease.

No doubt this new inspection station did play some role in reducing the threat of yellow fever. By identifying and detaining sick individuals, mosquitoes found fewer disease-carrying arms to feast on. But as with the sanitation measures, the architects of these measures misinterpreted their success. Public health officials were convinced that in draining swamps and low-lying areas, and in covering and/or improving sewer systems, they had eliminated the muck that bred toxic effluvia. And the managers of the Tinicum Island station believed that their elaborate processes were intercepting the disease before it reached the city. They remained divided on the exact reason for their seeming success as there was no consensus among them as to the cause or transmission of yellow fever. But rather than engaging in further debates, the Board of Health split the difference and appointed members from both camps. And consequently, while the contagionists on the board believed that by intercepting and detaining incoming vessels they were blocking the dangerous disease from entering the city, Rush's followers believed they were intercepting new sources of toxic miasma. Rush's followers worried less about the people than the cargos onboard. And just as he had blamed rotting coffee for the 1793 outbreak, his followers on the Board of Health were most suspicious of incoming shipments of coffee, as well as hides and rags. These were similarly susceptible to rot and consequently the production of yellow fever causing miasma.

Of course, the truth behind the city's improved health was more complex. Colder northern winters had always shortened the disease season; the first frosts killed the mosquito vector that carried the disease. And the public sanitation campaigns, while not ridding Philadelphia and other northern cities of toxic miasmas, did reduce mosquito habitats and therefore the breeding grounds for disease-carrying swarms. In the South, however, there was a different story. Warmer weather meant mosquitoes could more readily survive or lie dormant through colder seasons, providing a more robust vector population when the disease made its return. Compounding the problem, southern cities were far less aggressive in developing the sorts of sanitation programs that contributed to improved health conditions in the North.[7]

The failure of southern cities to pursue more robust sanitation measures was not because the disease represented a distant or only periodic threat. Between 1840 and 1860 not a year passed without the disease hitting at least one southern city. Whereas northern cities had escaped a major outbreak since 1825, Charleston, South Carolina; Norfolk, Virginia; Savannah, Georgia; Mobile, Alabama; and Pensacola, Florida, suffered regular epidemics. But no southern city faced more frequent or deadly epidemics than New Orleans. Located at the mouth of the Mississippi

River, the first American port of call for commercial vessels sailing from the West Indies, the simple combination of proximity and tonnage made it inevitable that crews or mosquitoes carrying yellow fever would reach New Orleans. Once offloaded, the disease could reach epidemic proportions thanks to the robust mosquito population luxuriating in the city's warm, damp climate.[8]

Locals anticipated some sort of yellow fever outbreak virtually every summer—but some summers were worse than others. The disease killed roughly 1,500 people in 1804, the same number in 1817. As many as 6,000 may have succumbed to the disease in 1819 and perhaps 8,000 in 1832–33. Yellow fever killed 12,000 New Orleans residents in 1853 and another 10,000 in the seven years leading up to the Civil War.[9]

But the extent of these yellow fever outbreaks was as much a consequence of culture as climate. In the first half of the nineteenth century there were extraordinary profits to be made in sugar and cotton. By the mid-1830s New Orleans recorded more export profits than any other city in the United States. And the commercial opportunities attracted migrants from all over the country—and the world. Between 1803 and 1860 more than a half-million white immigrants entered the United States through New Orleans. By 1840 the city was home to more than 100,000 people, individuals willing to risk the city's recurring epidemics in the belief that their hardiness, or luck, would earn them a big payday.[10]

New Orleans's boom conditions bred a transitory mindset that inhibited the growth of a more civic-minded leadership class—one that might have invested in public health and sanitation projects. Even more uniquely, New Orleans's business community actually adapted to yellow fever, weaving its regular appearance, deadly toll, and, for the lucky, consequent immunity into the city's social, political, and cultural fabric. Persons surviving yellow fever and "earning" the golden ticket of immunity—or "seasoning"—became privileged members of the community, preferred candidates for employment and promotions, bank loans, political office, and even marriage.

Of course, not all those who were supposedly immune received preferential treatment. Ironically and tragically, Black slaves who city leaders erroneously believed naturally immune to yellow fever did not see their conditions improve. Instead, Blacks' "immunity" made them all that much more valued as workers, leaving the city's merchants and public officials that much more committed to protecting the institution which lay at the heart of their profits.

Whether they adapted, turned a blind eye, or only periodically pursued modest public sanitation campaigns, southerners tended to accept the prevailing belief throughout the country that disease emanated from local filth. The vast majority of southern physicians agreed that yellow fever was born in the toxic effluvia bred in the putrefying animal and vegetable matter most often found in low-lying areas or squalid urban quarters.[11]

The South's leading medical journal, the *New Orleans Medical and Surgical Journal,* was not unwilling to publish a range of opinions on the origins of the disease and its dissemination. On its pages William G. Williams rejected the idea of local origins and argued that the disease was "indigenous to tropical latitudes and incapable of production beyond." But he conceded that he was "among the few" who believed this.[12] Far more agreed with P. H. Lewis, who in more than one article argued that yellow fever was spawned in local muck. In assessing Mobile's 1843 epidemic he stressed that the city was surrounded by swamps, and that its "deep, wet black alluvial" soil was a veritable animal graveyard. Contributing most to the city's toxic effluvia were the three hundred pounds of fish and eight hundred pounds of animal matter tossed daily into the streets to fester in the southern sun.[13]

Lewis was a particularly vehement defender of the miasmatic theories earlier championed by Rush and canonized in the pages of the *Medical Repository.* Lewis's attack on the "violent partisan contagionists" of New York intent on blaming foreign importation suggests that, at least for him, the etiological debate had not lost its combative edge.[14] But on the pages of the New Orleans journal he was far from alone. W. P. Hort echoed Lewis in suggesting that the greatest threat to the health of New Orleans residents was the filth collecting on the river's edge—"damaged flour, condemned fish and oysters, fruit, hay, hemp, rotten hides, potatoes, grain and dead animals."[15] And E. D. Fenner, in supporting the argument, took extra pains to show that the flow of troops through New

Orleans, going to or returning from the war in Mexico, were important only in that they represented an unacclimated disease target. True, yellow fever was raging in Vera Cruz, but there was no evidence of contagion or importation from that source. The disease was generated locally and then feasted on the unacclimated soldiers passing through the southern city.[16]

Just as Rush's eighteenth-century assessment persisted among southerners, so too did his therapeutic regimen—at least to an extent. J. Hampden Lewis noted that while bleeding was less commonly prescribed in New Orleans than in other southern towns, he himself routinely took twenty-four ounces of blood on a first visit to a yellow fever victim. Unless, of course, the patient seemed too frail; then he would turn to leeches. Forty applied to the anus would relieve the congestion of the stomach, liver, bowels, and even brains of a sufferer.[17]

T. A. Cooke was also an enthusiastic bleeder. He described taking as many as thirty ounces at an initial bleeding, and then another half-gallon within a few hours. The ninety ounces taken within the first day represented roughly half of the body's total supply.[18] J. F. Beugnot matched Rush's heroic posture as well as his therapeutic advice. Like Rush, Beugnot linked yellow fever to a "sur-excitation" of the body's vascular system that "nothing save the loss of blood" could calm. Moreover, this needed to be done quickly and aggressively. Just as the disease "runs its course rapidly," the physician needed to "keep pace with it." Echoing Rush's 1793 pronouncement that "intrepidity in the use of the lancet" was fatal, Beugnot concluded that "nothing is so dangerous as temporizing, which many physicians decorate with the false name of prudence."[19]

While most southern physicians clung to miasmatic explanations for the disease, and many employed the same depletion therapies popularized by Rush, they did offer an important riff on Rush's theory—one that impacted their response to the threat. As the disease spread to interior towns, they concluded that while the infecting agent could not be spread from person to person, it could be transported on certain goods or in the tainted air trapped in trunks and other containers.[20]

For example, when yellow fever struck Woodville, Mississippi, in 1844, the New Orleans Medical Society concluded that their ideas surrounding the disease needed to be examined "de novo." Located more than one hundred miles from New Orleans, fifteen miles from the Mississippi River, and at an elevation more than three hundred feet above its banks, the small town did not fit the topographical profile typically associated with the disease. It was not surrounded by swamps, and its residents did not live on crowded, poorly ventilated streets. The rainwater collected in cisterns and creeks remained "transparent and sweet," not foul and discolored. Yet in the late summer and fall of 1844 a reported 80 percent of the city's seven hundred residents contracted the disease, leading to sixty-three deaths.[21]

In looking for an answer to this atypical outbreak, a pair of physicians dispatched by the society to investigate conceded that there was no point in reviving ancient questions surrounding the character of the disease: "In its present state science is on this point impotent."[22] Nor were most physicians engaged in this reexamination willing to rethink their long-standing dismissal of contagionism. (J. C. Massie added a historical touch to the anti-contagionist position by tracing the discredited theory to Pope Paul III. Contagionism was nothing less than an antiscientific conspiracy perpetuated by the "Romish church."[23]) But these physicians were swayed by the evidence that the disease did reach the city in some fashion through the person of Reverend W. J. Thurber, who passed through the disease-infested city of Galveston on 30 June before reaching Woodville on 12 July already showing signs of yellow fever.[24]

Investigating physicians constructed an elaborate schematic of all subsequent cases, their proximity to Thurber's location, and all forms of contact, direct and indirect, with patient zero. Their conclusion was that while not contagious, some sort of "infection" was the source of the disease spread, and that the "focus of infection" was highly mobile. Visually rich accounts from other interior towns added clarity to the idea. T. A. Cooke, for example, described the keel boats carrying cargo from New Orleans to Opelousas, and the deadly consequences of opening crates and baggage from the fever-filled city. The toxic air trapped in stored linens and clothes supposedly killed more than one unsuspecting laborer.[25]

This "recognition" of the disease's transportability had a significant effect in shaping southern public health policy. Rather than invest efforts in draining swamps, removing debris, covering sewers, and cleaning water supplies, public officials proposed stronger restrictions on trade and travel during epidemics. It is true that most public health advocates coupled their belief in transportability to the idea that the transported toxin required a nurturing environment to survive—and this meant that quarantines should be complemented by sanitation efforts. Yet despite all this, neither was pursued with any real consistency. The "usual pattern," concluded one historian, was for health boards to "coalesce during an epidemic and then fade away after the threat had passed."[26]

Ultimately, despite this variation on northern analysis and response, southern physicians toed much the same etiological line dominating northern practice—with one notable exception. Josiah Nott's writing on the role of insects in the origins and dissemination of yellow fever was both distinctive and largely ignored. Given the proliferation of unconventional medical ideas circulating in the decades before the Civil War, it may not be surprising that his ideas would have been lost within the cacophony. But Nott's suggestion that yellow fever was a distinct disease, caused and/or carried in some fashion by minuscule insects, represented the closest thing to a correct assessment of the disease prior to the end of the century—and the closest thing to a germ-based theory of disease in the United States prior to the revolutionary, albeit imported, revelations of Louis Pasteur and Robert Koch. What separated Nott from his American contemporaries deserves a close look.

Nott introduced his ideas in an 1848 article published in the *New Orleans Medical and Surgical Journal*. He began by challenging existing yellow fever theories that lumped the disease among a bundle of hot weather diseases tied to "gaseous or molecular emanations from the earth's surface." Instead, he declared yellow fever a "disease sui generis" with an "inherent power of propagation" corresponding to the "peculiar habits and instincts of insects." He did not claim to be breaking any new ground. Swedish biologist Carl Linnaeus, German zoologist Christian Ehrenberg, and Sir Henry Holland, physician to both Charles Darwin and Queen Victoria, had made similar observations—but the self-evident truths of animalcular theories had been drowned out by the prevailing miasmatic orthodoxies. Yet the disease that had appeared so frequently in Mobile over the last decade did not correspond with any "appreciable meteorological changes." Nor could its peculiar patterns of dissemination be explained by any of the known laws of gases. On the other hand, the disease could be counted on to subside with the first frosts, only to be "animated by another summer's sun, which calls from their slumbering places the various insect tribes."[27]

The specificity within Nott's analysis has been exaggerated by many. Several historians and medical entomologists have suggested that he specifically identified the mosquito as the yellow fever vector. He did not. He merely included it among a list of many insects that were active at night and easily transported by the wind. Further, he was vague on the question of whether the unspecified disease-bearing insect was the vector or the actual producer of the poison. But he was adamant in denying the claims of contagionists, at least in their belief that the disease was conveyed directly through person-to-person contact. Instead, he argued that the "germ or materies morbi" of yellow fever was transportable by insects.[28]

Nott's argument tapped into older theories of disease that had hovered outside the mainstream of Western medical thought for centuries. Roman agricultural experts Marcus Terentius Varro and Lucius Junius Moderatus had warned against disease bearing "minute creatures which cannot be seen by the eyes, which float in the air and enter the body through the mouth and nose." And the plague that ravaged Europe during the Middle Ages—so sweeping and indiscriminate in its reach—had inspired renewed interest in these theories. Most medieval physicians clung to more conventional notions that disease was an individual affliction, the result of an individual body's failure to sustain humoral balance. And toxic effluvia emanating from the earth, not airborne animalcules, was most commonly identified as the trigger for this humoral imbalance. Yet aided by the recently developed microscope, some seventeenth-century theorists laid out a different explanation for the plague and disease more generally. Skin diseases like scabies had long been associated with the tiny, barely visible insects that emerged from the torturous blisters. And Giovanni Bonomo argued that his microscopical studies had allowed him to more clearly observe the tiny tortoise-shaped creature, which resided in clothing and sheets and was the source of the common ailment, not just its byproduct. August Hauptmann soon offered a far more sweeping conclusion based on his pioneering work with microscopes in 1650: "Minute and almost invisible animalcules are the cause of all deaths in men and animals."[29]

One might think that the scientific community would have rapidly embraced animalcular theories as the microscope was more widely employed—that the ability to actually see these possible agents of disease would have substituted the visible for the imagined in constructing theories of health and illness. But this is not what happened. Insect-based theories of disease were cast to the margins of disease theory, and the microscope, a seemingly invaluable research tool, was all but ignored for two centuries. This twin failure represents more than curious episodes in the history of science. It played a crucial role in the stagnation of disease theory and thus requires a careful review.

The microscope was a long time in coming.[30] The ancients recognized that objects could be magnified through transparent spherical containers filled with water. Francis Bacon played around with lenses in the thirteenth century, and eyeglasses were introduced at roughly the same time. But the first real, functioning microscopes (and telescopes) did not appear until the early seventeenth century. Most historians credit a Dutch lensmaker, Hans Janssen (and/or his son Sacharias), with developing the compound microscope. And over the next fifty years sporadic references to the tool appear in the notes of prominent figures like Galileo and Descartes. But during these years the telescope found a larger market. It had uses beyond the scientific, for example, in navigation and war. It was not until midcentury that any serious and systematic employment of the tool would occur. Yet over the next fifty years, microscope-wielding pioneers examined semen, blood, hair, fat, tears, and sweat, as well as protozoa, sponges, parasites, and crystals.

The most sustained work dealt with insects, culminating in the production of Robert Hooke's *Micrographia* in 1665. But it was Antonie van Leeuwenhoek, possibly the most important microscopist of the

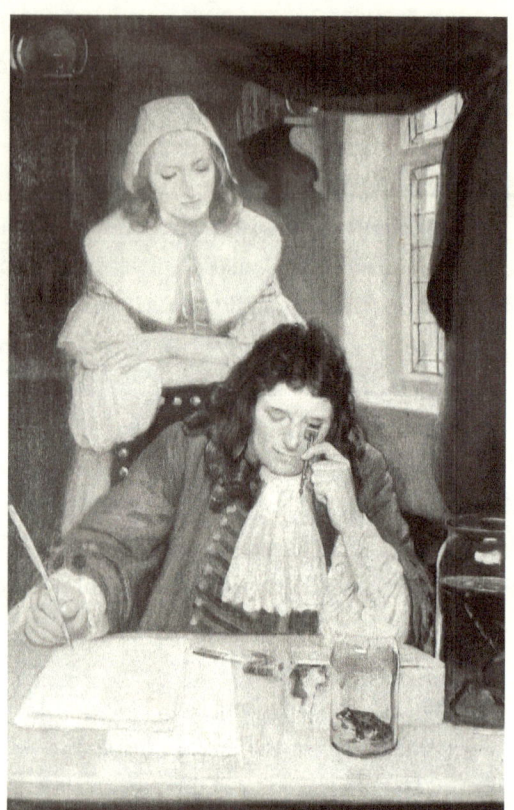

Antonie von Leeuwenhoek peering through the tiny lens of his handheld microscope, by Ernest Board, 1831. (Wellcome Collection)

era, who extended this study of tiny creatures to the even more tiny animalcules he first found in a tub of water. He described these as ten thousand times smaller than the tiny insects observed by other scientists with the naked eye, and he celebrated their variety with gusto—their tails and paws, their serpent-like appearance.

Hooke's work, in particular, increased interest in the microscope, both its scientific potential and voyeuristic possibilities. Collections of microscopist drawings were soon widely available on the continent. But by the early eighteenth century this initial interest had largely waned, in part because the primitive tool was so difficult to use. Most of the early models had to be handheld; the aperture was tiny, and consequently properly illuminating the subject was difficult.[31]

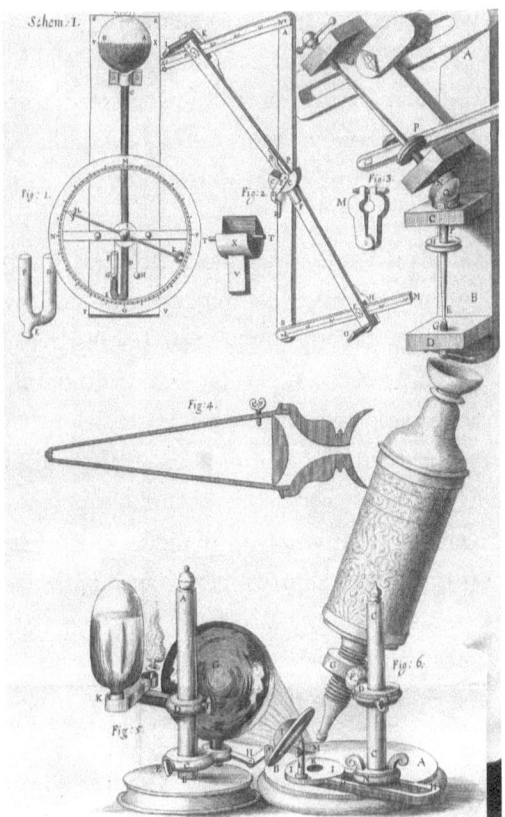

Robert Hooke's microscope. *Micrographia; or, Some Physiological Descriptions of Minute Bodies Made by Magnifying Glasses* (London: James Allestry and John Martyn, 1667). Hooke developed microscopes that were far superior to the first handheld instruments. (National Library of Medicine)

American scientists were among those showing little interest in the device. Harvard acquired a screw-barrel or double microscope in 1732; Yale purchased a compound microscope in 1734. But they were not incorporated in any significant way into either teaching or research, possibly because they were too hard to use and yielded images that could be terribly distorted. Even Hooke acknowledged that "it is exceedingly difficult in some objects to distinguish between a prominency and depression, between a shadow and a black stain, or a reflection and a whiteness in the color."[32]

For many historians, this neglect and eventual rediscovery of the microscope were simply a matter of developing more easily used and sophisticated instruments, like the Spencer Microscope developed in New

York in 1847, which boasted a wider angle of aperture and improved magnification.[33] But other historians have not been so willing to tie the lethargic embrace of the new technology to its imperfections. Instead, they have argued that the microscope's fate was tied more to the philosophical environment in which it was introduced and to one of the early scientific debates with which it became associated.

The critical figure in this analysis is Van Leeuwenhoek. The Dutch scientist inspired a school of followers with his wide-ranging studies of the microscopic animalcules he observed in water. But it was his discovery of spermatozoa that generated the most controversy—and ultimately suspicion—about the microscope. Van Leeuwenhoek was not alone in identifying what appeared to be minuscule flagellating animalcules within semen. And as others chimed in with their own details of the spermatozoa they observed through their microscopes, it was hard to ignore the possibility that they had something to do with reproduction. Once Nicholas Andry documented that they were found only in men of virile age (not young boys or old men), and once Van Leeuwenhoek discovered the tiny organisms in the fallopian tube of a female dog after mating, the case seemed settled.

But the exact part played by spermatozoa in reproduction was not. These discoveries occurred as philosophers and scientists vigorously debated the nature of generation. Most embraced some variation on epigenesis—the idea that plants and animals gradually develop the organs, internal systems, skeletal structures, and appendages that characterized the fully developed organism. For Aristotle, the material foundation of the organism was found in either the egg of the oviparous or the menstrual blood of the viviparous. But the developmental potential within this material was unbound by its contact with male semen. Once this occurred, the organism gradually assumed its implicit but not yet actualized form.

Two thousand years later, path-breaking anatomist William Harvey sought to remove much of the distinction that Aristotle drew between oviparous and viviparous creatures. While nothing so obvious as a chicken's egg could be found in women, he insisted that an egg, albeit unobservable, must exist within the uterus. And he also challenged Aristotle's claim that this material foundation of the future being was prompted into development through contact with semen. Instead, he argued that genesis was initiated by nothing so crude or mechanical. The egg was made fertile by a power more subtle and less corporeal. Fertilization was achieved by some power more analogous to a "ferment, vapouor, [or] odour." Yet, like Aristotle, Harvey concluded that organisms took form progressively, with first the heart and blood materializing, and only later the skeleton and head.[34]

Within a few years, Harvey's insight regarding the universality of a female egg to the process of generation was confirmed by other researchers. Dutch anatomist Regnier de Graaf claimed to actually find, not just hypothesize, eggs in a host of barnyard animals. And as a result, the theory that the ovaries of all female organisms produced eggs that made their way into the uterus where they became fertilized became widely accepted.

Yet even as these ovist theories acquired deeper support and sophistication, a different theory on the process of embryonic development challenged the dominant views of epigenesis. Proponents of "preformation" argued that organisms did not develop after implantation in the uterus; they simply grew. The entire organism—all of its organs, skeletal structures, and biological systems—existed within even its most minuscule forms. The organism did not evolve or elaborate, it merely expanded or unfolded over time. The most extreme version of the theory, contained within the idea of *emboîtement*, argued that all generations of animals, plants, and persons existed in complete but miniature forms within the bodies of their parents, who similarly existed in even more microscopic form within the bodies of their parents, where, like Russian nesting dolls, they patiently waited for millennia to be released.

The identification of spermatozoa within this intellectual environment created fascinating but also troubling possibilities. The aggressive, dynamic quality of the sperm, in comparison to the passive, inert character of an egg, suggested to many that its role, suggestively male, was the dominant one. But when incorporated within preformation theories the implications were disturbing. Nicolaas Hartsoeker suggested

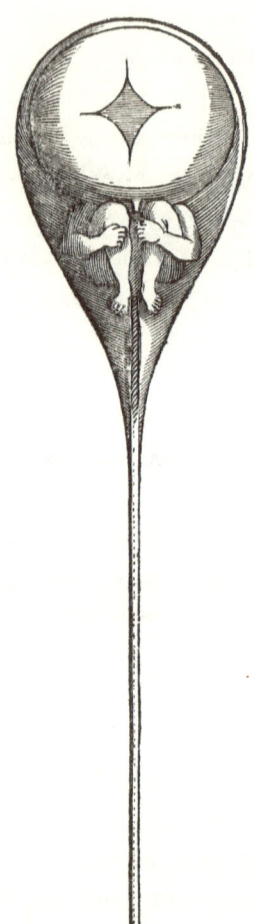

Pioneer microscopist Nicolaas Hartsoeker's drawing of the tiny humans contained within every sperm that he believed would be made visible by more powerful microscopes. Nicolaas Hartsoeker, *Essay de Dioptrique*, 1694. (Wellcome Collection)

that with proper magnification we might be able to detect human-like features inside the tiny spermatozoa—that within these flagellating organisms could be found, in fact, fully formed miniature humans waiting to implant themselves within the uterus and grow. Ethicists retreated in horror. What might this mean for all the millions of sperms discharged without finding a seat in the womb? How could this be reconciled with any theory of human beings, even the smallest, as soul-filled children of God?

The religious and ethical challenges surrounding spermatozoa—and preformation more especially—contributed to the uneasiness surrounding the microscope as a tool for serious scientific study. As most microscopists followed Hartsoeker's lead in claiming that their instruments affirmed both the existence and role of spermatozoa, as well as the truth of preformation, scientists and philosophers less wed to the instrument pulled back. By the end of the seventeenth century even some of its earlier celebrants, like Hooke, had lost faith in the microscope's ability to revolutionize scientific study. And students of other pioneers turned against their mentors. Even the followers of Italian microscopist Marcello Malpighi, who made extraordinary discoveries about the human circulatory and nervous systems, questioned the value of his preoccupation with anatomical structure. His microscope-aided examination of the body's organs and fluids, they argued, had yielded nothing of practical benefit, and "no solid advantage to medicine has proceeded from such studies."[35]

The instrument had faced an uphill battle from the start. It was introduced into a philosophical environment already skeptical about the idea that even instrument-enhanced vision could be a reliable source of information. Bacon had voiced a common belief that "the subtlety of nature" was greater than that of the "the senses and understanding." He was fascinated by the microscope but resigned to the belief that the real force or meanings within nature were more subtle and small than even the most powerful magnification. Others feared that the tool would provide misleading information—for example, a rough surface that through magnification appeared smooth. The technical limitations of the new devices only fed this skepticism. Within this contested environment, the fantastic claims of pioneers like Hartsoeker, who actually published a drawing of the fully formed mini-human he imagined encapsulated within a sperm, helped send the microscope to the shelf for the next two hundred years.[36]

Thus, by the mid-nineteenth century, when Nott published his animalcular ideas, several centuries of philosophical suspicion and technological skepticism had converged to inhibit their exploration. Animalcular theories of disease survived on only the edge of medical science on both continents. But there is something particularly curious about this fact for America in that American science was focused so closely during the early nineteenth century on natural science—its animals, plants, birds, and insects. There is no denying the odds stacked against the microscope and the suggestive animalcules it revealed. But given Americans' fascination with their continent, given their obsession with cataloging their natural wonders, it is surprising that a theory of disease that focused on the most populous of nature's inhabitants did not gain wider purchase—especially when these theories made appeals to principles that were central to early American thought: common sense, the observable within nature, and American exceptionalism.

A century before Nott, English botanist Richard Bradley was one of the few who tried to sustain the ancient theories of animalcular causation. In 1721 he suggested that the plague's recent reappearance in Marseilles was caused by "poisonous insects." More broadly he argued that "pestilential distempers" were spread by tiny airborne insects that were inhaled or ingested. These tiny insects were carried across entire continents by easterly winds, and once infecting an individual, the insects and their eggs could be transmitted from person to person through sneezing, coughing, or simply breathing.[37]

Bradley relied on the microscope in building his theory, but in making his argument he appealed more to common sense and shared observations of nature. He reminded readers that eighteenth-century life taught that insects or worms, most likely inhaled or ingested, could live in and thrive within the human body. And farmers had for centuries operated under the premise that the blights that attacked their crops were caused by airborne insects—that is why they stoked smoky fires to ward off flying pests. Nature also offered hints to explain the selective nature of these insect-triggered epidemics. Just as insects had specific nesting patterns, they most likely targeted specific individuals who emitted a certain odor. Animals and humans weakened by poor diet emitted a certain effluvia, Bradley said, that attracted disease-carrying pests. And once anchored within even a small segment of the community, these toxic insects—or perhaps it was their eggs—could be rapidly and broadly disseminated because of their tiny size through the simple act of breathing or sneezing. Bradley's theory even explained the effectiveness of certain age-old folk remedies like tobacco smoke and other aromatics: they provided an odiferous antidote to the smells that drew the disease-carrying insect to the vulnerable victim.

English physician Henry Holland, writing a century later, made a similar appeal to the known and observable in nature. The natural world offered dozens of examples of poison and pain-wielding insects from bees to ants and spiders. How hard was it to imagine that among the thousands of minute animalcules, there might be some "capable of acting as a virus on the human body?" While some might scoff at the idea that something so tiny could devastate entire continents, Holland speculated that "their power of morbidity" might exist "in some ratio to their multitude and minuteness." Holland turned to the recent cholera epidemics as proof. The disease had followed an irregular course, leapfrogging some communities as it traveled before infecting others more distant. Its outbreak in various communities was not preceded by similar climatological patterns or atmospheric conditions. There was no evidence of other sorts of "natural morbid" causes such as gas or mineral exhalations. On the other hand, the irregular, unpredictable behavior of epidemics did match the behavior of insect swarms that come, stay, go, and even die off inexplicably.[38]

John Crawford, Baltimore physician and professor of natural history at the University of Maryland, was the first American academic to advance an animalcular theory of disease. In a series of articles published in 1807 he reminded readers of the predatory behavior of insects like the ubiquitous louse. Most revealing for Crawford was the ichneumon, the "common leveller," which attacked a huge range of insects, laying their eggs on the bodies of their victims, their larvae devouring their host on hatching. Was it not likely, he argued, that humans would be subject to the same attacks—"the plague, yellow and every other fever, and every other disease . . . occasioned by eggs insinuated, without our knowledge into our bodies?"[39]

While to an extent, Crawford could appeal to Americans' shared experience, in order to make the leap from insect-insect predation to insect-human attacks he had to ask his readers to embrace a rather large premise. With little evidence to support his idea that human skin was covered with minuscule insect eggs, he asked his readers to accept the idea that each organism "comes into existence, is nourished and terminates its being in a way remarkably similar." He conceded that this comparison of insects and humans "might appear humbling" to our "lofty pretensions," but he was adamant that "the cause of death in any one species must be the same in every other."[40]

The effrontery within the premise may explain why Crawford's ideas gained few followers. Thirty years later John L. Riddell, professor of chemistry at the College of Louisiana, offered an animalcular theory of disease that was more palatable and actually closer to the truth. Like Bradley and Holland, he buttressed his argument with evidence provided by nature. But he also appealed to his American audience's iconoclastic instincts in calling for the repudiation of ideas dating to "the dark ages of science." In an 1836 address, he argued that the "matter" of contagions and harmful miasmas was of an "organized nature" and consequently subject to the "same general laws . . . of animal or vegetable bodies." This "matter," which he variously described as "corpuscles," "miasmatic molecules," and "infusory animalcules," sat at the "lower confines of organic nature," yet, like other organic entities, possessed the ability to propagate. This ability rendered these organic carriers of disease more dangerous than ordinary, inorganic poisons, as their degree of morbidity was not determined by the amount of contact, that is, "the smallest possible quantity is adequate to the production of the greatest possible effect." The result was that deadly disease could be conveyed by "wingless beings, of transcendent minuteness . . . on the wings of the wind to the most remote regions of the earth."[41]

Eight years later, Josiah Nott similarly prefaced his animalcular theories with a critique of the inherited "delusions" that plagued Western medicine. Complaining that "it takes almost as much time to uproot a false medical doctrine as a false religion," he outlined the self-evident facts about yellow fever that should demonstrate to any observer the flaws within both contagionist and miasmatic theories. The disease did not necessarily appear near shipping or commerce; it did not always surface near stagnant pools or putrefying waste. There was no easy correlation between the disease and the weather nor did its spread follow any sort of pattern, at times moving rapidly, at others slowly and methodically from house to house "as would a tax collector." The only clue to the origins and behavior of the disease, Nott concluded, was found in the mysterious but commonly observed behavior of insect swarms.[42]

Nott pulled back from blaming insects—both visible and microscopic—for all major diseases, but he did note that Ehrenberg had successfully shown that "living, dead, or fossil animalcula" filled "every breath of air we breathe, every particle of fluid or solid we swallow, all the water of the land and of the sea, every solid of the earth we tread upon."[43]

Nott's suggestion might have been tempered and he might have couched this introduction to his theory within an appeal to Americans' common sense and their contempt for religious and intellectual traditionalism, but still he found few supporters—even among early American entomologists, including those who had identified the threat posed by some insects.

Thaddeus William Harris wrote in 1842 that the destructive power of certain species was widely acknowledged by New England farmers. Yet separating Harris from Nott was the former's discussion of predatory insect species within a plea for what a later century would label biological control. The centuries-old preoccupation with insects' harmful potential blinded us, Harris argued, to their value within nature. Moreover, their destructive threat was triggered by the destruction of their natural habitats and removal of their natural predators. Foreign commerce had also led to the introduction of nonindigenous, and thus hard to manage species. The answer lay in more careful study of insects' natural history and management techniques sensitive to the "balance originally existing between plants and insects, and between the latter and other animals."[44]

Harris's emphasis on the generally benign impact of insects reflected the celebratory tone struck by his predecessor, Thomas Say, within his landmark taxonomy of American insects. Say's work was the product of some of the grand exploratory projects of the early republic. Born in 1787, the son of a Philadelphia Quaker physician, he joined an expedition into Florida sponsored by the Academy of Natural Science in 1817. The trip was something of a disappointment. Returning to Philadelphia in May 1818, before the insect-filled summer months, Say discovered few unfamiliar species. But in 1819 Say set off again, this time as the chief naturalist for an expedition into the American West led by Stephen Long. Departing from Pittsburg in May, the corps traveled down the Ohio River to the Mississippi and the Missouri Rivers before heading off by horseback to the Rockies. In 1823 Say set out again with Long, this time up the Minnesota River and across the Great Lakes. The insects Say observed and documented in these travels became the foundation for his seminal *American Entomology*.[45]

Like James Audubon, whose path crossed Say's in 1819, Say was anxious to present America's natural kingdom. But he was inspired even more by Thomas Jefferson's crusade to celebrate the abundance and vigor of the country's natural kingdom. While Jefferson searched for proof of a living mastodon, Say cataloged the variety within American insects as part of a collective rebuttal to the French Comte de Buffon, who had mocked the strength and diversity of the flora and fauna within the American continent.

Say's nationalism was perhaps most apparent in his insistence that American insects be named by American entomologists. He was furious when American naturalist John Le Conte shipped a cache of beetles to Paris to be identified and named by French naturalists. But Say was also a self-conscious scientist, intent on advancing the profession as much as America's reputation. He insisted that exploratory expeditions move beyond the haphazard methods of Lewis and Clark; America's scientific community demanded more than simply the "barren narration of the existence of a rock here, a tree there, of a singular unknown animal, etc." Instead, the naturalist must offer more on "the nature of that rock, tree, or animal, its affinities, uses, etc." Say's call for the professionalization of natural science was important, but he interpreted his own counsel somewhat narrowly, limiting his efforts to taxonomy and cataloging. Between 1817 and 1828 he published three volumes of *American Entomology* and identified even more insects in scientific journals, yet only on a few occasions—noteworthy for their rarity—did he move beyond very exacting and precise descriptions of insect anatomy.[46]

Later students may have been frustrated by Say's failure to record insects' behavior and significance. But the rationale behind Say's limited agenda was provided in the preface to the first abbreviated version of *American Entomology* published in 1817: "Each shell, each crawling insect, holds a rank important in the plan of Him, who fram'd this scale of beings." As Say's biographer explained more fully, his goal as a naturalist was defined by his belief in the great chain of being—his assumption that God's created order could be arranged along a "long unbreakable chain stretching from the lowest to the highest form." The most pressing unresolved question was where each creature should be placed along that chain.[47]

Say's cosmological assumptions did more than narrow his research agenda—they also influenced his assessment of the insects he studied. He was not willfully blind to the negative impact certain insects had on agriculture. *Aegeria exitiosa* was a "silent, insidious destroyer of the peach tree." Locusts destroyed crops, and once gorged, the "putrid exhalations from their dead bodies [produced] pestilence in the train of a general famine which is the consequences of their voracity." But Say was more ready to point out the wonderful harmony within nature, as evidenced by the wasps that reduced the threat of the Lepidoptera by eating their larvae, or even more in the behavior of many Hymenoptera that live "harmoniously in large communities . . . laboring for the attainment of the common object." Written while living in New Harmony, Robert Owen's short-lived attempt at building a classless communalistic society, Say's celebration of the bee was offered as "proof of intelligence" sufficient to "render insecure the distinction . . . between the blindness of instinct and the splendid nature of reason."[48]

That Say never pushed beyond his taxonomic efforts, that he never inquired into the larger possibilities lying within the field he was pioneering, that in elevating the subject of entomology he never took a sustained look at theories of animalcular disease causation, may be explained by both his scientific priorities as well as his sense of God's creation. Reflecting the post-Calvinist evangelicalism that was coming to dominate American religious orthodoxy, Say's sense of nature orderly and balanced, a manifestation of God's beneficent design, was incompatible with animalcular theories that made nature's most abundant and diverse inhabitants the sources of so much suffering.

But Josiah Nott was willing to go where Say was not. His view of nature and the cosmos was very different.

Nott was always something of an iconoclast, or perhaps more precisely a selective iconoclast. His father, Abraham, had been born in the North and attended Yale, yet he built a thriving legal practice in Columbia, South Carolina, while accumulating property and slaves upcountry. Josiah consequently grew up sharing many of the traditional values held by the state's slaveholding elite. Yet when he enrolled at South Carolina College in 1822, he was drawn to the religious skepticism of the school's controversial president Thomas Cooper. Cooper, even though English-born and Oxford-educated, was, like Nott, comfortable with southern slavery, yet he was an outspoken critic of organized religion and challenged the authority of the Bible. When attacked by the state's Presbyterian leaders, Cooper responded with an eloquent defense of intellectual freedom and the primacy of scientific truth that resonated with the college's freethinking students. For Nott, Cooper's strident anticlericalism and attacks on biblical authority, his affirmation of science, and his vigorous defense of slavery and states'-rights provided something of an intellectual template.[49]

The combination of the conventional and anticonventional was most fully expressed in Nott's racial views. During the 1840s and 1850s, Nott became a leading proponent of the belief that whites and Blacks, while united as members of the same genus *Homo*, were different species. This argument represented the maturation of a set of ideas—actually, two sets of ideas—that had been percolating among American intellectuals for a half-century before crystalizing within a "scientific" defense of slavery.

The first of these was rooted in medical concepts dating back decades. When Benjamin Rush pleaded with Philadelphia's Black leaders to recruit caregivers from their community under the impression that Blacks were immune to the disease, he drew on an idea advanced by John Lining during South Carolina's yellow fever epidemic in 1748. Within just weeks, amid evidence that "the Negroes are everywhere submitting to this disorder," Rush would recant this position. But this concession was lost within the increasingly more popular view that there were physiological and anatomical—and thus medical—differences between white and Black bodies.[50]

Rush's change of heart revealed not just an intellectual flexibility but also the ways that ideas about race were informed by larger intellectual constructs—and politics. With increasing frequency Rush would argue that any observed differences between Blacks and whites in terms of disease susceptibility could be explained less by race than by condition. If Blacks were more vulnerable to illnesses, he argued, it was due to the physically and morally degrading conditions of slavery.

Rush was ardently opposed to slavery; for ten years he served as president of the Philadelphia Abolitionist Society. In a striking illustration of his ability to merge medical science and political philosophy he argued that slavery, and more broadly the lack of freedom, was a debilitating stimulus. Similar to depression or melancholy, it possessed the power to undermine the more healthful stimuli on which the body depended, thus causing disease. Rush's belief in the physiologically debilitating power of slavery eventually reached an even more extreme conclusion. During the 1790s he argued that even skin color was a morbid condition caused by disease, and perhaps reversible through freedom.

When Rush first raised this possibility, he suggested that leprosy might be the root cause of the African's color. But later in life his belief in skin's mutability seemed to converge with his belief in the debilitating effects of slavery and the healthful effects of liberty to suggest that once freed, once converted from slave to yeoman farmer, the Black person's health—and skin color—would change. Rush's fascination with Henry Moss—a former slave who seemed to be "turning white" the longer he enjoyed freedom—was tied to this belief that skin color and social condition went hand in hand.[51]

But Rush was somewhat atypical. More physicians and scientists, in both the North and the South, persisted in the belief that the differing medical responses of Blacks and whites were connected to permanently differing physiologies. Over the course of the antebellum period, this view would grow, due largely to southern physicians interested in advancing their professional and financial interests.[52]

As slave populations grew, and with the termination of the international slave trade in 1808, southern planters took an increased interest in protecting the health of their valuable labor supply. In response, southern physicians recognized that both their prestige and fortunes would grow if they could present themselves to these planters as experts on the distinctive health needs of enslaved people. In other words, while their arguments might eventually serve slavery apologists interested in establishing the physiological and mental differences between the races, in the short run these physicians were more interested in establishing their ability to provide the specialized—and lucrative—medical care that planters' Black labor force required.

The profits within this sort of specialized practice extended beyond preserving the health and fitness of a planter's enslaved workers. Physicians assumed more elaborate roles within the institution as "experts" verifying and testifying to the "soundness" of slaves. Physicians were routinely hired to inspect slaves being sold and issue certificates of soundness based on these examinations. They might be asked to provide expert testimony in court if a buyer believed they had been defrauded. Or they might be hired to conduct a medical examination as a prerequisite to an insurance policy being issued to protect the slaveowner's investment.[53]

This emphasis on the physiological differences between white and Black bodies bumped into something of a contradiction when southern medical schools began using deceased slaves for dissection. Anxious to recruit more northern students, southern schools promised easier access to bodies—albeit Black bodies—for study. Clearly, the benefits for prospective students rested on the premise that physiologically Black and white bodies were essentially the same. There was no value in studying or dissecting a Black body if the lessons learned could not be applied to the white patients these northern students hoped to court.[54] But the financial considerations of both southern physicians hoping to build practices and southern medical schools hoping to increase enrollment wasted little time on this intellectual inconsistency. And as a result, the idea of physiological difference gained increasing purchase among southern physicians.

At the same time, a second set of ideas drawn from a handful of overlapping "scientific" disciplines provided additional "proof" for the physiological basis of race. Various ideas regarding racial differentiation were voiced from multiple quarters in the eighteenth century, yet most of these were embedded in a "monogenetic" theory of human origins—that is, even if racially divergent, both Blacks and whites could trace their origins to a common pair. For these students of race, religious orthodoxy—the universal parentage of Adam and Eve—could be preserved by attributing racial difference to environmental factors. But during the eighteenth century, challenges to this comfortable accommodation grew. Some expressed skepticism that the environment—climate, geography—could work such dramatic changes within the timeframe typically associated with human occupancy of the earth. Others simply said the stark differences between the two races defied any attempts to tie them to the same originating pair. Instead, these more radical theorists cautiously attempted to replace the monogenetic explanation of human origin with a "polygenetic" account that suggested the different races must be, in some fashion, rooted in different creative moments, different originating locations, even different original pairs.

During the early nineteenth century these polygenetic theories were given "scientific" support through several interrelated disciplines—craniology, anthropometry, phrenology—that used the meticulous measurement and comparison of skulls to reach a predictable set of conclusions about the comparative intelligence of different races. The foremost American scholars engaged in this analysis were Charles Caldwell and Samuel George Morton. Morton's 1839 *Crania Americana* was especially important in advancing the idea that differences among the races were fixed. Based primarily on the comparison of skulls that he had collected from all over the world, and reenforced by his study of the political and cultural achievements of different races, he concluded that the races could be situated on a tidy hierarchy, with whites situated at the top.

But for all his scholarly rigor, Morton sidestepped the religious implications of his work. While arguing that the differences among the races were fixed, he steadfastly avoided speculating on the relationship between these fixed differences and the biblical account in Genesis that suggested all humanity could be traced to a single pair. Yet one of Morton's most ardent admirers was not nearly so timid. Josiah Nott, like most

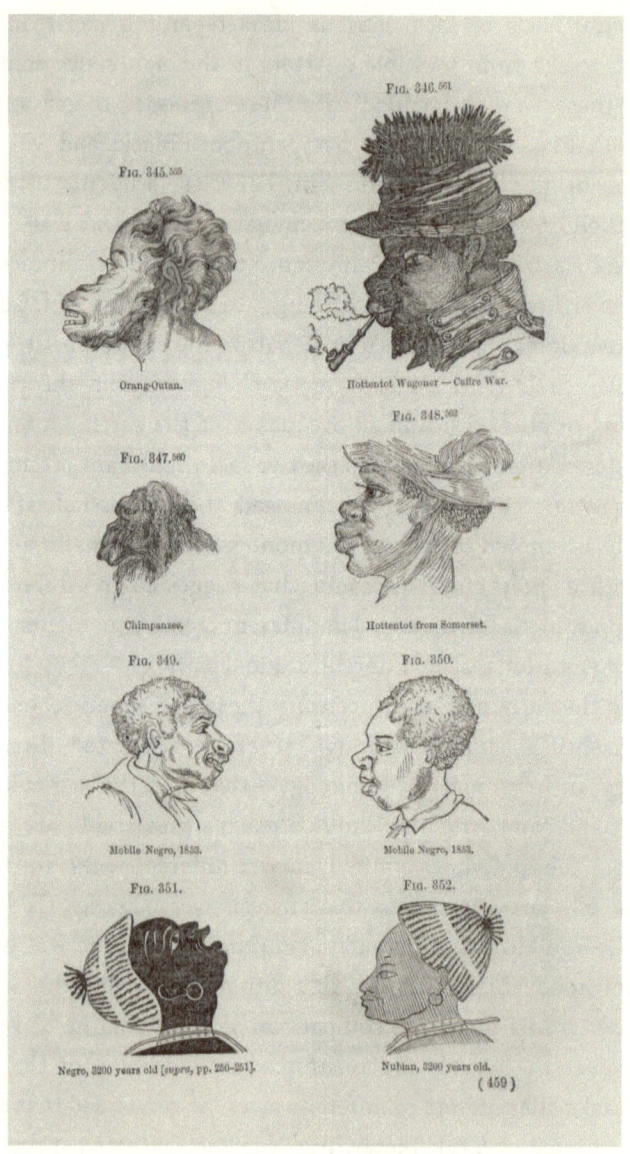

Josiah Nott's racial hierarchy, from Nott and George R. Gliddon, *Types of Mankind; or, Ethnological Researches Based Upon the Ancient Monuments, Paintings, Sculptures, and Crania of Races*, 8th edition (Philadelphia: J. B. Lippincott, 1860). Nott used facial and cranial comparisons to argue for the superiority of the white race and suggest that African features were similar to those of chimpanzees and orangutans. (Wellcome Collection)

Fig. 339. — Apollo Belvidere.⁵⁵³

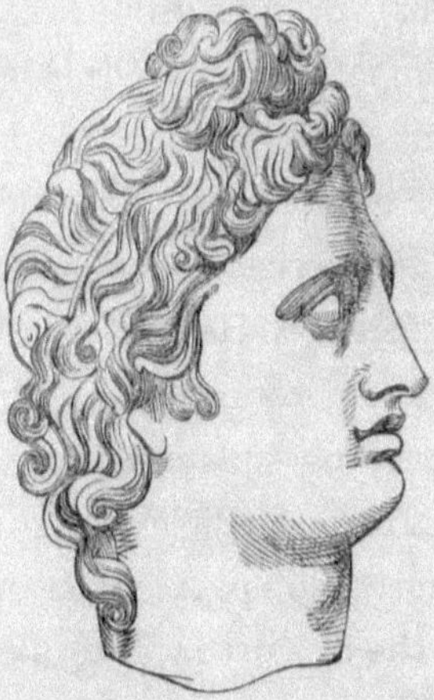

Fig. 340.⁵⁵⁶

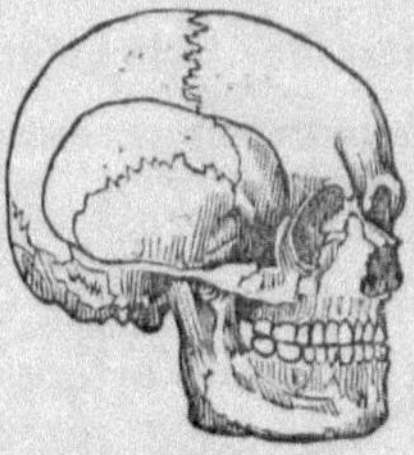

Greek.

Fig. 341. — Negro.⁵⁵⁴

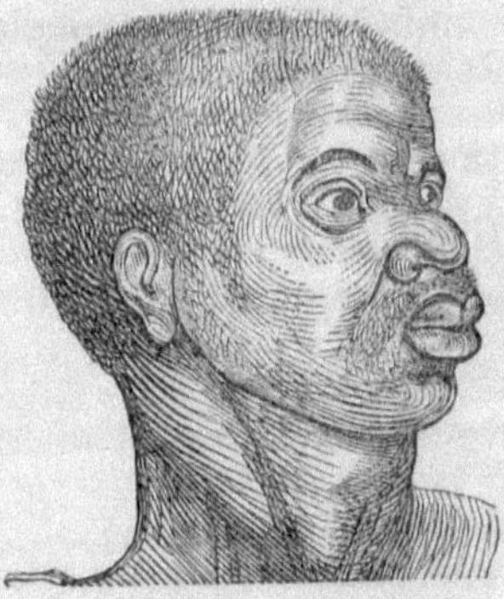

Fig. 342.³⁵⁷

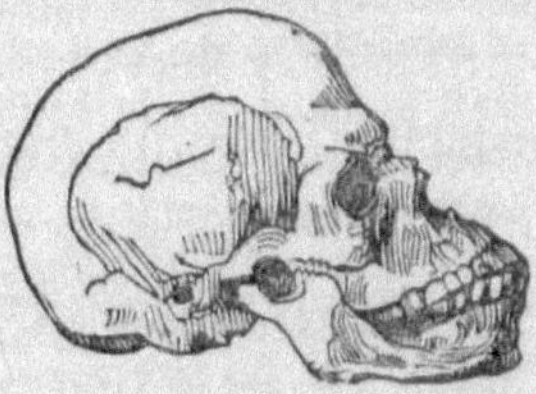

Creole Negro.

Fig. 343. — Young Chimpanzee.⁵⁵⁵

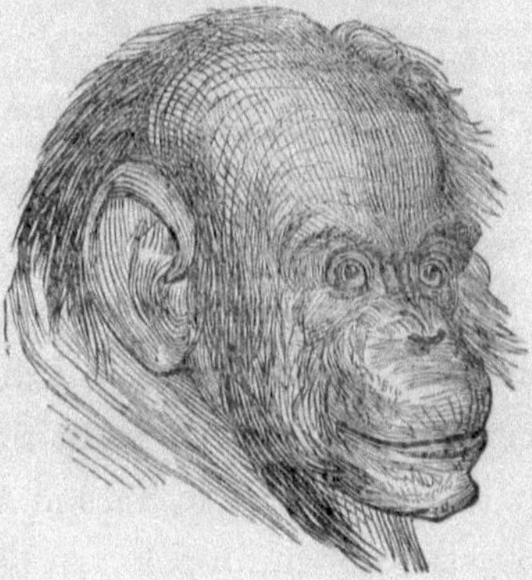

Fig. 344.⁵⁵⁸

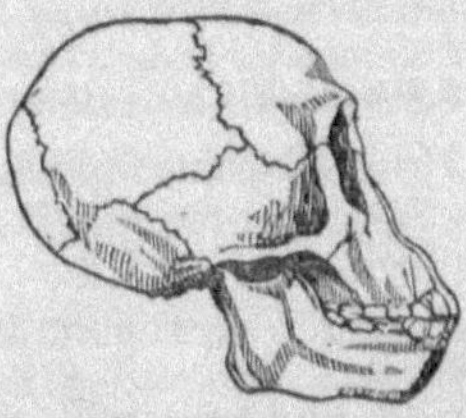

Young Chimpanzee.

(458)

southerners, embraced Morton's belief that the racial differences were fixed and hierarchical—a critical premise within the growing slavery apologetic that labeled slavery a "paternal" practice protecting Blacks from barbarism in Africa and ruthless competition in the free-labor markets of the North.[55] But where Nott separated himself from Morton and most southerners was in his willingness to embrace the religious implications within Morton's views—his willingness to challenge religious orthodoxy in explaining the origins of these differences. He scoffed at those attributing racial differences to climate and environment; he refused to make peace with religious orthodoxy by accepting explanations for racial differences that others found in various parts of the Bible: God's curse on Cain or perhaps Ham, the separation of the world's people after the effrontery of Babel. Instead, Nott argued that the distinct races resulted from distinct creative moments. Blacks and whites were not descendants of the same original pair; they sprang from different founding couples, only one of which was introduced in Genesis.[56]

As attractive as Nott's racial ideas were to many southerners, this attack on biblical authority, on the orthodox understanding of human creation, was troubling. He tried to argue that he did not entirely discount Genesis—he only suggested that its account of creation was incomplete, explaining only *one* of God's creative moments. Nature offered proof of periodic temporal catastrophes—floods, fires, an ice age—that had gone unchronicled in the Bible but had been followed, Nott argued, by additional creative moments.

To his critics, Nott's claim that he was not challenging fundamental bases of Christianity was unconvincing. As his argument unfolded, the accepted timetable of Mosaic creation also fell under the scythe of recent science. The meticulous calculations of James Ussher, Anglican archbishop and biblical scholar, which placed Adam and Eve in the garden in 4004 BC, were disproven, argued Nott, by the discovery of the Rosetta Stone, which had opened up ancient Egyptian texts. Furthermore, botanists had recently discovered six-thousand-year-old trees in Africa and Central America. And the skull collections of anthropologists like George Morton, with whom Nott developed a close relationship, offered physical "proof" of the fixed differences among the races.

Nott was no atheist; he argued that there was a divine intelligence at work in the universe. Distinct species were introduced by an "all-wise creator" into the climates and environments best-suited to their physical and mental characteristics. Even the destruction visited on the earth periodically reflected a constructive intention: "The organized tribes in existence have more than once perished to make room for a new order of beings.... These epochs or revolutions in nature ... [were] accompanied or preceded by inundations and other catastrophes." But biology and human nature could also make war against this progressive divine trajectory. Nott fretted over the self-destructive, actually species-destructive refusal among whites to avoid sexual interaction with Blacks, joining other racial theorists before him in waxing apocalyptic over the danger posed by miscegenation. People of mixed race, Nott suggested, sitting somewhere in between whites and Blacks on the racial ladder, were inherently defective. Either sterile or of feeble virility, they represented a "degenerate, unnatural offspring, doomed by nature to work out its own destruction." Virtually every southerner, Nott claimed, knew that those of mixed-race were more prone to disease and shorter-lived than both whites and Blacks. That is why, Nott argued, if one hundred white men and one hundred Black women were placed on an island, both would eventually become extinct. As proof of the supposedly fatal dangers within miscegenation, Nott pointed out that the proud Egyptians—who, he claimed, were originally white—had seen their civilization subverted through imperial success. In conquering the Ethiopians, they had taken on a destructive "black stain, both moral and physical."[57]

Nor, Nott added, could whites reverse the apocalyptic dangers within miscegenation through philanthropy. The white conquest of Central and South America only offered evidence of the futility of attempting to elevate Indigenous people. And history had similarly demonstrated that Blacks, like American Indians, according to Nott, the lowest of the human species, could not be educated or civilized: "All the powers of earth cannot elevate them beyond their destiny."[58]

Unlike Thomas Say, who believed that the cosmos was divinely ordered and filled with a multitude of creatures which, without exception, attested to God's beneficent design, Nott's universe was filled with human beings who waged war against God's progressive purposes and insects that launched epidemics. For Nott, history was scarred by periodic convulsions, catastrophic events that destroyed peoples and communities while introducing different, and biologically threatening, new races. His was a world in which the insect kingdom—filled with the most abundant, diverse, and ubiquitous of God's creations—was characterized less by the ecologically balancing behavior of the wasp or the intelligence of the bee than the swarms that behaved unpredictably and irrationally, without any recognizable logic or design, spreading disease and death.

Today Josiah Nott is perceived as a man of intellectual contradictions—archaic and bigoted in his racial views yet insightful, perhaps even prophetic, in his understanding of disease. His polygenetic ideas are condemned for their racist and transparently political motivations, the intellectual underpinnings of a dying economic system, not the product of any sort of serious scientific exploration. Yet his rejection of miasmatic and contagionist theories, theories that had dominated the etiological landscape since the founding of the republic, and his recovery and advance of marginalized animalcular theories of disease are recognized by many as the most viable understanding of yellow fever reached in America prior to the emergence of germ theory three decades later. Yet while contradictory to modern sensibilities and values, they were united in Nott's mind, tied together within an understanding of biology and history.

And it is this seemingly contradictory combination of ideas, in some ways consistent with and in others repugnant to modern sensibilities, that poses the real challenge to students of American ideas and our understanding of intellectual progress. Nott's recovery of unpopular ideas about animalcular causation did not spring from an unequivocally progressive mind. The determinative trait shaping his thought was not a commitment to rational or scientific thought but rather a willingness to think—albeit selectively—beyond orthodoxies in religion as well as science—his willingness to cast aside prevailing notions of creation and the cosmos, his willingness to challenge popular ideas about the benign nature of God's creation and the unalterably progressive direction of history that had become widely held elements within antebellum American ideology. And the willingness of various constituencies to only selectively embrace elements of his thought—the southerner who could accept his racist ideas but not his religious, the northerner who could embrace part of his racial ideology but not his sense of the violence implicit within the natural order or the potentially catastrophic direction of history—suggests that the full range of Nott's theories could not find wider purchase because they demanded too many departures from important elements within American thought outside medicine.

Nott died in 1873 on the eve of the European discoveries that would transform medicine. His understanding of disease would be validated. Yet, in his own mind, so too was his understanding of history. In the years following the Civil War, he believed he saw the cataclysmic consequences of racial mixing, the foolishness of all attempts to elevate inferior races, and the civilization-destroying results of abolishing slavery. With the South defeated, and the reformist agenda of Radical Republicans "tragically" transforming, if only temporarily, the South's political and social order, his warnings of the potential for humans to sabotage the progressive designs of an "all-wise creator" seemed realized.

Probably nothing galled him more than to see the medical school he had established in Mobile converted by the Freedmen's Bureau into a school for recently freed slaves. For Nott, the simultaneous transformation of medical science and southern society would have offered proof that he was right in both his medical and racial-historical theories. Today, we recognize in these events evidence of what he got right as well as what he got wrong.

9

After a Century the Mystery Is Solved

THE ANIMALCULAR THEORIES OF disease advanced by Josiah Nott in the decades preceding the Civil War would not be widely embraced. Instead, most physicians clung to the same ideas about miasmas that had shaped their responses to the medical crises of 1793 and 1832. And consequently, when Americans confronted their next medical crisis in 1861, the therapies first applied in the camp and on the battlefield were little changed from those applied decades earlier.

Yet it would be wrong to say that medicine and the medical profession did not evolve at all during these years. Examined from another angle, a lot did change, especially during the quarter-century prior to the war. For example, the number of medical schools increased significantly between 1800 and 1860. In 1800 there were only four medical schools in the United States. There were thirteen in 1820, thirty in 1840, and forty-seven by 1860. And most of this expansion occurred in the South and West. As access to formal medical education increased, so too did the "standard" method of professional preparation. By the second quarter of the century, medical school had replaced apprenticeship as the dominant path toward medical practice.[1]

But this institutional growth should not be read as professional advancement. The vast majority of these schools were proprietary and not affiliated with any college or university. Instead, they were the creation—often short-lived—of a handful of practicing physicians who saw the financial rewards of founding and running a school as superior to the vagaries of a private practice. A physician turned professor or administrator could make as much as five times the average physician's salary.

Moreover, as these schools needed to attract students, their survival required concessions to the market. This meant that entrance requirements were generally low if not nonexistent altogether. And lax admissions standards were coupled to lax degree requirements and unambitious pedagogy. Difficult subjects like Latin and physics were dropped from the curriculum, along with written exams and the preparation of a thesis. Most schools demanded that some sort of clinical preparation under the supervision of a preceptor be pursued alongside coursework, but by 1850 the traditional three-year standard was demanded by only four of the thirty medical schools in operation. And seven schools did not require any apprenticeship at all.[2]

Even though intellectually suspect, a degree from a proprietary school provided access to the profession. And consequently, most of the more established schools—those affiliated with colleges or universities—found that they had to follow suit and relax their own admission and degree requirements. At the University of Michigan, only 14 of 350 medical students possessed a college degree on admission to the medical school in 1871. At Harvard, only 19 percent of those admitted to the medical school during the same period arrived with college degrees. One administrator complained that more than half of the students could not even write.[3]

During these years the course of study leading to a medical degree acquired some consistency. Students took two four-month terms—the second being a repetition of the first. And they typically took courses in chemistry, materia medica, anatomy, physiology, and surgery. This standardization of curriculum corresponded with a standardization of medical theory and therapeutics. As more and more physicians accessed the profession through medical school rather than apprenticeship, miasmatic theories of disease became further entrenched. But just as noteworthy is what they did not study. Pathology would not become a central part of medical education until the second half of the century when an interest in cellular pathology gathered more attention along with increased use of the microscope. (Prior to the Civil War, the vast majority of medical students never used a microscope.) And while students did study anatomy, many, probably most, explored the body exclusively through lectures—without access to labs or cadavers for dissection.

The inability of medical school to provide a consistent supply of cadavers for dissection was tied to popular opposition to the practice that was codified in state and local laws. But as medical schools proliferated, faculty and students put increased pressure on state governments to revise these laws, especially since knowledge of human anatomy was increasingly seen as the distinguishing characteristic of the medical profession—the body of knowledge that separated the "trained" physician from the poorly prepared practitioner.[4]

But in the face of this rising professional pressure, large portions of the public offered steady resistance. Not surprisingly, the loudest protests came from those whose bodies were most likely to end up on the dissection table. The poor, immigrants, Blacks, and transients made up a hugely disproportionate percentage of all bodies taken, legally or not. Medical students and professors, or commercial "resurrectionists," usually began their search in potters' fields, where families or local officials were less able or willing to provide protection to the recently buried. Some families tried: They carefully arranged flowers, stones, and trinkets around graves in an attempt to detect an intruder, or buried their loved one's body so deep that it could not be unearthed in a single night.[5]

Importantly, members of the middle class were often just as vocal in their opposition to the removal and dissection of bodies. For many, their objections were religious. Those maintaining orthodox beliefs in the resurrection of the body recoiled at the idea of defiling the bodies that would be summoned to the judgment seat at the end of time. And for many, this religious revulsion was coupled to a broader cultural celebration of "the beautiful death" spread through sentimental fiction and didactic tracks. Over the course of the nineteenth century, families spent increasingly large sums on funerals and burials—events that would turn a person's death into an opportunity to tell the story of their commendable life. Elaborate grave markers and coffins, eulogies, songs, poems, and even souvenirs for funeral attendees were part of elaborate celebrations of the good life and beautiful death.[6]

This moral and religious opposition to human dissection was reflected in the structure of the earliest anatomy acts that allowed only the bodies of criminals executed for capital crimes to be turned over for dissection. In 1784 New York authorized judges to turn over the bodies of people executed for murder, arson, or burglary, while in 1805 Massachusetts added an exclamation point to its law against dueling by stipulating that persons executed for dueling could be turned over as well. But pressure from medical schools and physicians led the Massachusetts legislature to pass a less-restrictive anatomy act in 1831. Under its terms, any body left unclaimed, and thus to be buried at the public expense, could be surrendered for study and dissection, provided the deceased had not expressly requested burial. A couple of other states followed suit—Connecticut in 1833 and New Hampshire in 1834. But within a decade, renewed public pressure led to their repeal. Only Massachusetts and New York, which passed the "Bone Bill" in 1854, allowing the unclaimed bodies of vagrants to be turned over for dissection, had anatomy acts on the books at midcentury.[7]

But these legal obstacles did not bring anatomical study to a complete end. Medical students and their teachers were not above raiding the local graveyard. And for the more timid, there were many underground sources. Prison officials who employed a loose interpretation of the statutes allowing for the sale of bodies of capital offenders were one source. Another was professional robbers who were willing to risk the legal penalties given the considerable profits to be made. During the 1820s a skilled craftsman who earned roughly twenty-five dollars a week working his trade could get the same amount for a freshly buried body. The business was lucrative enough that even persons with professions and historic names were willing to join—Dr. John Revere, son of the legendary patriot, arranged a shipment of bodies from New York to Boston for Harvard's medical students.[8]

These clandestine efforts were justified as necessary to the advance of science and the cultivation of the skills necessary to perform the noble work of saving lives. But many historians have argued that the acquisition and dissection of bodies was also part of a ritual, an initiation of sorts into a fraternity, bound together not just by the possession of distinctive anatomical knowledge but also by daring schemes, midnight adventures in the graveyard, or negotiations with an illegal vendor before late-night dissections behind closed curtains and locked doors.[9]

Most likely, the truth behind it all is a mixture of both—medical students did gain some knowledge of the body but they did so through a rite of passage that separated them from others while uniting them through an extralegal experience as well as a body of esoteric knowledge. Whether students gained more serviceable knowledge dissecting a rapidly rotting body than they did studying texts or the wax models imported from Italy is unclear. As it putrefied, a corpse's muscles would tighten and lose their natural texture and plasticity, organs would shrink and become discolored. And the odors—overwhelming for more than one anatomical explorer—were so foul that they deterred prolonged or close inspection.[10]

While it is impossible to say how many medical students actually benefited from dissecting a human body, it is clear that one area of instruction that did grow during these years was obstetrics. In 1800 only two of the nation's four schools included obstetrics within the course of study. But over the next fifty years obstetrical instruction became part of the core curriculum and professors dedicated to the subject were added to medical departments. The expansion reflected a fundamental fact about medical education: a barrier to reform was the absence of new knowledge. Reformers had a hard time rethinking the content and structure of medical education so long as there was so little new medical knowledge to add to the course of study. But in the field of obstetrics, a handful of achievements encouraged its expanded place in the curriculum. The introduction of anesthetics and their use in delivery and new understandings of puerperal sepsis represented important new content for dissemination. Educators also gained appreciation for the value of "demonstrative midwifery." Over the second quarter of the century an increasing number of students participated in a delivery during their course of study. In addition, by midcentury physicians were not uncommonly performing successful ovariotomies and repairing vaginal fistulae.[11]

The dearth of new medical information and the stagnation of American medical science meant that most of the reform movements launched before the Civil War focused on little more than the structure of medical education. Reformers suggested that the terms of study be extended, that admission to medical study follow the taking of a college degree, and that formal apprenticeships be required of all taking the M.D. But there was far less discussion of the curricular content or methods of instruction—little discussion of the value of labs and clinical observation, no significant reassessment of the course content leading to the degree.

The inadequacies of an American medical education were among the first issues addressed by the American Medical Association when it formed in 1847. A survey of nineteen American medical colleges made clear just how poorly they compared to European schools. Simply put, American medical students spent less time studying fewer subjects than their European peers. American students could complete a degree in as little as two years—French, Austrian, and German schools required three and a half to four years of study. European students also spent far more time in clinical observation and were required to conduct dissections. Most American students did not have access to similar clinical experiences and only five of the nineteen American schools surveyed made anatomical dissections a requirement for the degree.[12]

America's simpler path to the profession allowed far more aspiring physicians to enter practice. The report estimated there were forty thousand medical school graduates practicing in the United States—or one for every five hundred residents. And when the long list of irregular practitioners "who swarm like locusts in every part of the country" were added to the count, it became clear why the profession was held in such low esteem and physicians found it so difficult to command reasonable fees.[13]

The report concluded with a call for "a uniform and elevated standard of requirements" for the M.D. degree. But even while doing so, the report's writers acknowledged that they could not demand too much in the short term. Most schools did not have the faculty to support a widening of the curriculum, and many schools were not affiliated with or had access to a hospital that would allow students to gain important clinical experience. As a result, the committee's recommendations fell far short of the standards set by France and Germany. And subsequent follow-up studies found that even these relaxed ambitions went largely ignored over the next two decades.[14]

To compensate for the inadequacies of an American medical education an increasing number of American students traveled to Europe to broaden their study. But there was an important change within this practice in the second quarter of the nineteenth century. Whereas earlier American students had tended to study in Leiden or Edinburgh, more and more chose France. The dismantling of the ancien régime had led to a more creative and democratic spirit within the French medical community. There were expanded opportunities through the elimination of the old medical faculties and, more importantly, a new approach to medical education. "Bedside teaching" was probably introduced in Padua, but in Paris it became the primary form of instruction. Collected within the city's network of hospitals, patients were examined through new techniques—percussion, auscultation—with their symptoms and therapies cataloged for comparative assessment. This "numerical" method, most commonly associated with Pierre Charles Alexander Louis, placed a premium on observation over experimentation; eschewing theoretical speculation for the statistical analysis of disease and therapy, practitioners compiled the natural histories of various diseases without getting lost in speculation over root causes. Perhaps most importantly, these studies were facilitated by French government policies that made cadavers easily available for dissection.[15]

Between 1820 and 1861 more than seven hundred Americans pursued professional improvement in Paris. Their purposes varied. While a small portion pursued a degree (fewer than fifty), more sought to add depth to their American studies—add the "Parisian polish" that might boost their professional profiles and marketability. In addition, many practicing physicians viewed the pilgrimage as a sort of sabbatical, time away from their practices (and families) to indulge in scientific study. In this regard, many expressed excitement at learning at the cutting edge of medical science. Decades earlier, Napoléon Bonaparte, hoping to win international respect, had declared access to the lectures and demonstrations offered throughout the city free to foreigners, leading American visitors to luxuriate in the opportunities for study—until the language challenges often dampened their spirits. But that being said, the vast majority of those traveling to France most commonly emphasized less the purely intellectual attractions than the rewards gained through practical experience. With cadavers readily available for just a few francs, American students and physicians could study anatomy in ways that were far more difficult to achieve back home.[16]

These opportunities for hands-on anatomical study, coupled to the more general emphasis on empirical study, were most frequently celebrated in the letters these travelers sent home. No doubt the pragmatism within this approach to medical science resonated with the collapsing confidence in deductive analysis expressed most forcefully during the cholera crisis of the 1830s. For the American medical community, divided by etiological debates, exhausted by partisan squabbles, and demoralized by its inability to simply comprehend the diseases that plagued them, this strictly empirical approach to medical study made sense. If physicians could not sort out the root causes of diseases, they could at least construct a more finely nuanced summary of the characteristics of these ailments and, through the compilation and statistical analysis of various therapeutic approaches, come to some sort of authoritative guide to best practices.

As a result, many returned to the United States committed to spreading the French system at home. They represented only a tiny fraction of the nation's practitioners and students, but the very fact of their travel reflected that they were not bread-and-butter physicians. Many came from privileged backgrounds, and many taught at medical schools or edited or contributed to medical journals. In other words, despite their small numbers they had the potential to exert an outsized influence. And indeed, many took a messianic interest in spreading the French forms of patient examination and medical education. They encouraged a greater commitment to clinical education and the adoption of the numerical approach to diagnosis and therapy.

But ultimately, their ability to transfer all that they had experienced was limited by the realities of the American environment. Opportunities for clinical study were restricted by the shortage of hospitals. State governments imposed severe restrictions on the collection of bodies and dissections. Even efforts to change the nature of their own practice proved difficult. Despite the lofty ambitions they brought home, few were able to overcome the limitations within the American medical community, and few managed to build practices similar to those they had observed in France.[17]

The bottom line is that when Americans encountered their next great medical crisis—the Civil War—the students graduating from America's medical schools brought much the same knowledge and practices applied in 1793 and 1832. Bleeding was less common, but purging was routine. Using the same rationale that made these therapeutics seem logical to eighteenth-century Americans, military physicians on both sides of the conflict purged, as one historian has argued, "until something immediately visible happened." In fact, one of the medical controversies during the war surrounded the recommendation made by Union surgeon general William Hammond that calomel be removed from the military drug chest. Physicians who had relied on the mercury purgative for years protested, contributing to Hammond's short tenure in office.[18]

Surgeons in the field did have access to the anesthetics developed in the 1840s. Ether's mind-altering properties had been recognized for over a century. During the 1830s experimental partygoers enjoyed the inhibition-loosening consequences of inhaling the liquid's fumes. Curiosity seekers paid money to see their neighbors act foolishly at county fairs while the more "scientifically minded" attended lectures and demonstrations at community centers. But it was a pair of dentists who began to actually explore ether's pain-reducing qualities. The most disciplined of these, William Thomas Green Morton, spent the better part of 1846 experimenting with the most effective way to deliver the vapors; his work culminated in a successful demonstration of a pain-free surgical procedure before a crowd of physicians and medical students at the Massachusetts General Hospital.[19]

By the Civil War, ether and chloroform were widely used to desensitize patients before surgery. And so, contrary to popular images of battlefield amputations performed with only whiskey to dull the pain, both anesthetics were widely used by Union and Confederate surgeons. Chloroform seems to have been used more frequently. It could be made to work more quickly and was not flammable like ether. Both agents were more readily available to northern doctors as they were produced in northern states and could be imported from Britain. But Confederate troops succeeded in raiding northern supply depots, and by mid-war a plant in Columbia, South Carolina, had begun producing sulphuric ether. One study estimated more than 120,000 uses of ether in treating battlefield wounds.[20]

But unfortunately only a few doctors seemed to recognize the relationship between sanitation and infection. It is true that both Union and Confederate physicians did introduce some lifesaving practices—but they did so without really recognizing how these innovations might be reducing the rates of infection. For example, believing that the foul stench in field hospitals contributed to the formation of dangerous miasma, Union physicians ordered the wards cleansed with a variety of chemicals such as bromine, carbolic acid, and iodine. These may not have purified the air in the way that physicians hoped, but they almost certainly reduced the volume of infection-carrying microbes. And while northern surgeons spread disease by sopping the blood of several patients with the same sponge, southern surgeons were forced to find an alternative due to the shortage of this basic surgical tool. They found one in cotton rags, and even raw cotton, which could not be reused so easily and could only be cleaned—and unknowingly sanitized—through submersion in boiling water. But for the most part, poor understanding of the link between sanitation and infection had horrific consequences. Amputees were often forced to undergo a second amputation, inches above the first, to remove the infected matter that set in along the edges of the first stump. And even with these repeat procedures, roughly one of four amputations resulted in death; when close to the torso, the death rate surpassed one in three. A chest wound led to death more often than not. Abdominal wounds had a survival rate of only 13 percent.[21]

Throughout the war, Confederate physicians faced the greater challenge. While Union physicians quickly recognized the value of distributing daily doses of quinine to their troops to combat malaria, Confederate doctors were unable to procure a steady supply of the wonder drug. The more general shortage of conventional pharmaceuticals led Confederate physicians to cautiously accept some of the botanicals promoted by the irregular physicians they had previously spurned, including Georgia bark—an antimalarial alternative to quinine. Yet still, Confederate doctors faced

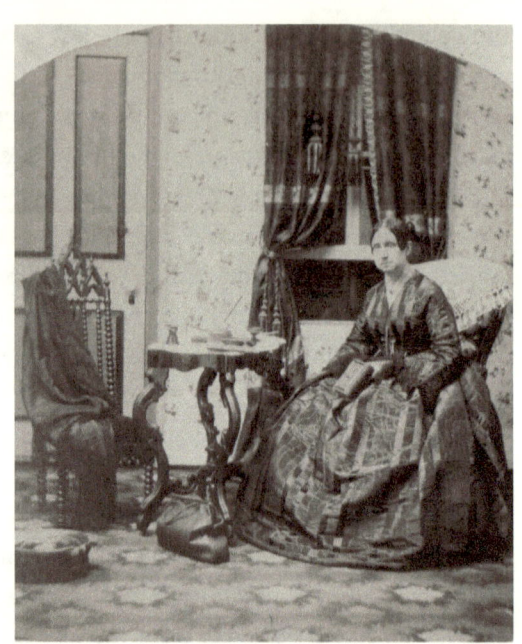

Dorothea Dix, Washington, D.C., August 1865. As superintendent of Union Army nurses, she hired more than three thousand to serve in general hospitals. The "homestyle" medical care they provided possibly contributed more to improved mortality rates than any wartime pharmaceutical or surgical innovation. (Library of Congress, https//www.loc.gov/item/2019630777/)

the more difficult task—especially given the Union Army's widespread use of the minié ball. Named after its designer, Claude-Étienne Minié, the soft lead conical projectile spread on contact, splintering bones and ripping larger tears in the flesh than conventional musket balls. As one Union surgeon noted, "The minié ball striking a bone does not permit much debate about amputation."[22]

On both sides of the conflict, physicians and administrators strived to improve their medical corps. Conscientious northern administrators took steps to improve ambulance services and camp hygiene, Dorothea Dix successfully campaigned for the integration of women nurses, and Jonathan Letterman improved and standardized the supply of medical supplies to the front. These innovations were not insignificant. In particular, attempts to deliver quality "home-like care" to injured soldiers confined to northern general hospitals led to survival rates far better than those achieved during the Mexican-American War. (The ratio of disease to battlefield deaths during the Civil War was two to one; during the Mexican-American War it was seven to one.) These efforts were tied to a military-based calculation: if injured soldiers were granted medical furloughs to return home where they might receive better care while rehabilitating, high desertion rates seemed likely. So, officials resolved to reduce that threat by providing more standardized care in the general hospitals established to treat the injured.[23]

But for the most part, these higher survival rates were tied to better nursing—keeping patients hydrated and well fed, changing bandages and linen more frequently—rather than more effective drugs or the application of more innovative therapies. In fact, a commitment to conventional medical theories shaped Surgeon General Hammond's efforts to expand and improve the hospitals he hoped would more quickly return wounded soldiers to their regiments. He personally oversaw the design of the new hospitals he commissioned, insisting that the wards be large and airy, and that each patient be given 1,200 cubic feet of space. Still believing that disease and infection were transmitted by corrupted air, not any sort of germ or discrete organism, he required that his hospitals be only one story, so that the toxic emanations from the sick and wounded would not rise and infect patients quartered on upper floors. There is no doubting the value inherent in practicing better hygiene, but the medical ideas informing his hospital design were the same ancient theories of disease floating around since Galen.[24]

Throughout the war Union medical officials remained so committed to traditional, conventional therapeutics that they barred irregular physicians from taking the surgeon's exam and entering their ranks. That was unfortunate, as greater receptivity to certain irregular theories might have contributed to healthier troops. When Alfred Hamilton succeeded in hiding his hydropathic training and securing an appointment to the 148th Pennsylvania Volunteers, he immediately set about applying hydropathy's sanitation principles in cleaning up the camp. The result was a measurable improvement in the regiment's health. But not every irregular physician was as successful in hiding his educational background. Other unconventional physicians were discharged from the medical service when their backgrounds were discovered.[25]

Pathbreaking medical historian Richard Harrison Shryock, writing roughly a century after the war's end, lamented that the persistence of ancient ideas and the failure to advance significantly beyond the analyses and therapeutics of America's earlier medical crises led to staggering mortality rates. He conceded that wartime physicians developed more sophisticated surgical skills and many became more skeptical about the benefits of bleeding. But the persistence of miasmatic theories of disease and the heavy reliance on purgatives and emetics took a deadly toll. Fairly comprehensive statistics compiled by the Union Medical Corps would seem to support these conclusions: 63 percent of all Union fatalities were due to disease, 12 percent were linked to infection following wounds or surgery, and only 19 percent were classified as battlefield fatalities. Confederate records are far less complete, but it is estimated that disease and infection accounted for roughly 65 percent of all troop deaths.[26]

Yet more recent scholarship has suggested that we should, at least partially, rethink this assessment. Even though they brought to their wartime service dated ideas, some military physicians, especially Union ones, used the experience to launch a revolution of sorts within American medicine. Leading this effort was US Surgeon General William Hammond. Professor of anatomy and physiology at the University of Maryland, he brought to his appointment extensive experience in laboratory research and a commitment to advancing the science of medicine. And he joined others in recognizing the opportunities within the sheer scope of the medical crisis, the range and volume of injury and illness caused by the war, to gather data and explore theoretical and therapeutic possibilities.[27]

To advance this objective, in 1862 Hammond issued Circular no. 2, which called for the formation of the Army Medical Museum as a repository for the case reports and "specimens of morbid anatomy" military physicians were ordered to forward from the field. Joseph Woodward, curator of the new museum, brought a similar academic and research-oriented background to his role, including extensive work in microscopy. Sharing Hammond's vision for the research and educational possibilities within the war, he aggressively pursued all seemingly relevant materials—amputated limbs, diseased organs—and when these materials were slow in arriving, he traveled to the front himself where he exhumed bodies to be hauled back to Washington for preservation and study.[28]

These materials, and the ambition behind their collection, fostered a new type of inquiry, and even rethinking of older ideas. As Woodward set about studying the camp-devastating incidents of dysentery and diarrhea, he urged field physicians to go beyond the natural-history approach of earlier researchers, who looked for environmental and seasonal correlations. Instead, he explored the impact of the diseases on the colon and bowels, microscopically examining the changes to the cells and colorectal tissues produced by these ailments. In a similar way, Woodward and others engaged in elaborate and fruitful studies of gangrene and erysipelas, experimenting with different chemical agents like permanganate, turpentine, and most successfully bromine to check the spread of these hospital plagues.[29]

In neither case were Civil War physicians able to draw the larger connections between the microscopic organisms they observed and the diseases they caused—the achievements of the period should not be overstated. For example, for all his work and even success, Woodward resisted all suggestions that the diseases he studied might be traced to some invading organism. But as he and others collected specimens and moved beyond the cataloging of symptoms to the analysis of tissues and fluids—doing so through more extensive use of the microscope—they tiptoed toward an understanding of the role of experimentation in advancing medical science. And while not wholly abandoning miasmatic theories, many began to view diseases as discrete entities, specific ailments with their own specific causes, "things" that were in some way contagious, not varied reactions to a common morbid force. As they collected materials for study and shared the observations drawn from research through journals like the *Medical and Surgical History of the War of the Rebellion*, they began to construct an intellectual and institutional infrastructure better prepared to receive and build on the bacteriological discoveries that would revolutionize medicine in the last quarter of the century.[30]

Yellow fever did not make a major appearance during the Civil War. New Orleans had suffered one of its regular outbreaks a few years before the firing on Fort Sumter. This 1853 outbreak was a particularly deadly one, killing an estimated eleven thousand people, more than 7 percent of the city's population. Another two thousand died in an epidemic that hit Norfolk, Virginia, two years later. Yet the worst fears of northern officials never materialized. The US Sanitary Commission prepared a detailed report in 1862 outlining how the Union Army Medical Corps should deal with any outbreak that might occur while occupying a southern city. It summarized the mushy hybrid that had formulated around the disease sixty years earlier. Yellow fever was the product of a toxic miasma, but the safest course was to maintain quarantines just in case it might arrive via ship. While the disease was unlikely to be conveyed through contact with victims, it could be transmitted through bedding and clothes. In other words, the conversation had advanced little. Fortunately for Union military and health officials, the catastrophe they feared never occurred—despite the prayers of southerners for a deadly visitation on the invading army.[31]

Following the war, epidemics returned to New Orleans in 1867 and 1873. And in 1878, as word of German researcher Robert Koch's discoveries about anthrax began to spread across the United States, a major epidemic swept through New Orleans and up the Mississippi. One observer suggested that more than 200,000 people took flight as the disease stormed through Vicksburg and then Memphis. An estimated 120,000 people sickened; about 20,000 died. But the reaction to the disease, while differing regionally, revealed that the fundamental questions had not changed. While northerners tended to blame local filth and urge sanitation programs, southerners emphasized its transportation via goods on commercial vessels, and thus relied on quarantines for their safety. And the robust debates about treatment that had accompanied the 1793 epidemic were replaced by the fatalism that had greeted cholera's arrival. One Memphis doctor admitted that he could do nothing more than serve as "a practical pilot . . . with an intimate knowledge of the channel along which he must guide and direct this human float." The American Public Health Association was forward-thinking enough to call for a national investigation of the deadly epidemic. But the keynote speaker at the association's 1879 meeting offered a shockingly dated summary of human disease: "These pestilences indicate the various deep-seated wrongs and neglects, vices and sins of the people. Whenever the human race is in such situation as to lose its strength, courage, liberty, wisdom and [lofty] emotion, the plague, cholera, and fever comes."[32]

The inertia crippling American medicine more generally had been put on graphic display just a few years earlier at the International Medical Conference held as part of the Philadelphia Centennial Exposition. Among those speaking was Joseph Lister, the Edinburgh physician and professor whose research had revealed the benefits of antiseptic surgery. In a packed lecture hall, he described the dangers to a surgical patient posed by dust and airborne bacteria and demonstrated the proper methods for sterilizing surgical tools and even the surgeon's own hands. No doubt many were inspired by Lister's lesson, but conference attendees also received a very different message when they passed through the US hospital building on the exposition grounds. There, Thomas Eakins's newest painting, *The Gross Clinic*—intended to pay homage to American medical progress—captured the far-from-sterile methods of the American surgical theater. In the painting, Samuel Gross, Philadelphia's most prominent surgeon, strikes a professorial pose while his students and/or fellow physicians dig—ungloved and ungowned—into the thigh of a young patient.[33]

In a final piece of irony, Lister and Gross were seated alongside one another at the congress's closing dinner. Perhaps event planners were hoping for some intellectual fireworks. Gross had recently written that "little, if any, faith is placed by any enlightened or experienced surgeon on this side of the Atlantic, in the so-called treatment of Professor Lister." Yet Lister would have the final say. While his methods quickly revolutionized surgical procedures, Gross's skepticism and Eakins's painting offer powerful illustrations of the lethargy that continued to plague American medicine.[34]

Yet while most American physicians remained stuck in place, European researchers were busy turning medical science on its head. Robert Koch's positive identification of the bacterium responsible for anthrax in 1876 did not occur in a vacuum. His work built on the seminal advancements of other European scientists. Lister's recognition of the danger to surgical

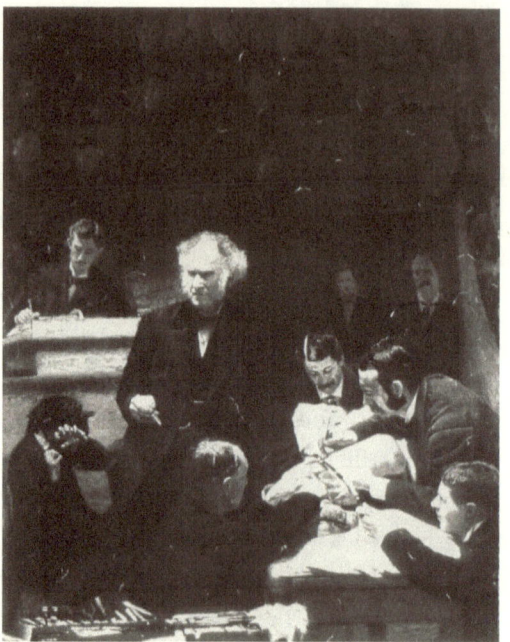

The Gross Clinic, by Thomas Eakins, 1875. Eakins intended to honor surgeon Samuel Gross in this painting. Followers of the British physician Joseph Lister were horrified by the ungloved, ungowned, nonsterile procedure. (National Library of Medicine)

patients posed by airborne microorganisms had followed Louis Pasteur's studies of putrefaction and fermentation. These studies debunked ancient theories of spontaneous generation by demonstrating that neither could occur without the introduction of microorganisms—an organic substance isolated within a sealed, sterilized container would neither putrefy nor ferment.[35]

Even the specific bacterium responsible for anthrax—*Bacillus anthracis*—had been identified years before Koch turned his attention to the disease. Two French researchers, Casimir Davaine and Aloys Pollender, had described certain rod-shaped bacteria in the blood of diseased cattle, and Davaine had further established that infusions of blood from a sick to a healthy animal would trigger the illness. But they could not explain how animals could succumb to the disease by merely grazing in a pasture that had contained sick animals years earlier. Koch solved the mystery by recognizing that there was a spore stage in the lifecycle of the responsible bacterium. These spores could lie dormant in the soil, surviving freezing winters and searing summers, before launching another deadly epidemic years after the diseased animals had been removed.[36]

Koch drew on other technological achievements in advancing an emerging germ theory of disease. Rapidly improving photomicroscopy and bacteria staining methods enabled him to better visually capture the microorganisms at work. And his success in developing methods for isolating these microbes within a pure culture provided the last piece in the formulation of the "postulates" that would guide bacteriological research for decades.[37]

Previously, attempts to positively identify a specific bacterium as the responsible agent of a specific disease had been stymied by the inability to isolate the suspected agent from other microorganisms. Koch recognized that the rod-shaped *Bacillus anthracis* could not be absolutely proven as the cause of anthrax until it could be separated from the surrounding flora and inserted into a healthy test subject. Koch's experiments, initially with boiled potatoes and eventually with a nutrient gelatin, enabled him to cultivate mediums on which he could create pure cultures for not only anthrax but also tuberculosis.[38]

The critical second of his four postulates that would guide further research was now a practical reality. To establish the microbial agent responsible for a specific disease he argued that the researcher must (1) observe the suspected agent in abundance in a diseased animal or person, (2) isolate the agent and grow it within a pure culture, (3) introduce the isolated suspect into a healthy subject, and (4) observe the existence of the suspected microorganism within the now diseased subject.[39]

Guided by these postulates and utilizing these new methods, European researchers commenced a systematic effort to identify the discrete microorganism that triggered individual diseases. And while scientists in the Americas played little role in this initial game-changing research, they did eventually contribute significantly to the unmasking of yellow fever's mysteries.

Juan Carlos Finlay was born in Cuba in 1833. The son of a Scottish physician, Finlay studied medicine at Jefferson Medical College in

Philadelphia before setting up practice in Havana. Interested in yellow fever, he was appointed by the Spanish governor to serve as a liaison to the US Yellow Fever Commission in 1879. By 1881 he had concluded that the spread of the disease was explained by neither contagionist nor miasmatic theories. Instead, some sort of vector was required, and soon his search was focused on the mosquito. His conclusion did not occur in a vacuum. A French physician, Louis-Daniel Beauperthuy, had suggested decades earlier that mosquitoes might be spreading the disease by transporting minuscule pieces of rotting toxic matter that they injected while biting a victim. And in China, Patrick Manson had discovered that mosquitoes transmitted the tiny worm responsible for elephantiasis. But still, Finlay's conclusions were largely rejected during the 1880s, only to be revived by researchers following the Spanish American War.[40]

Yellow fever and other tropical diseases like malaria had long been the scourge of European armies in the Caribbean. The army Napoléon dispatched to quell slave revolts in Saint-Domingue was decimated by yellow fever—an estimated fifty thousand French soldiers and sailors were killed by disease with yellow fever taking the far greatest toll. A century later, Spanish troops trying to smash an independence movement in Cuba met a similar fate. Between 1895 and 1898 Spanish official documents recorded more than sixteen thousand troop deaths due to yellow fever. But it has been argued that officials chronically underreported disease fatalities; one estimate suggests a more accurate tally of yellow fever deaths would surpass thirty thousand. Beyond fatalities, in the last year of the war, only 55,000 of a total Spanish force of 230,000 were healthy enough to fight.[41]

The disease crippling the Spanish Army was a contributing factor in Americans' decision to enter the war in support of the revolutionaries. For decades, it had been widely argued that many of the recurring yellow fever outbreaks on American soil could be traced to Cuban sources. But after the devastating epidemic of 1878, this argument gained momentum—even the ship supposedly responsible for the fever's introduction in New Orleans was identified. Other factors contributed to the belief that addressing Cuba's yellow fever problem was critical to reducing the threat posed by the disease to the United States. A Senate committee on immigration reported that 100,000 persons traveled back and forth between the United

States and Cuba annually. Plans for the construction of a canal across Central America meant that Cuba would become an even more important depot in American commerce, and in 1895 Surgeon General Walter Wyman concluded that sixteen of the nineteen epidemics hitting America since 1862 had originated in Havana. When yet another yellow fever epidemic striking New Orleans and other southern communities in 1897 was traced to Cuba, policy and opinion makers were more insistent that the only solution was for the United States to seize Cuba and launch sanitation campaigns aimed at ridding the island of the threatening disease. As the *Houston Daily Post* argued, "If annexing Cuba will result in eradicating yellow fever . . . by all means let us annex it at once."[42]

The proposal was double-edged. While there might be eventual health benefits, in the short term American intervention would mean exposing American troops to the deadly scourge. Yet after American troops did enter the war in 1898 in support of the revolutionaries, they managed to end their "splendid little war," as one US official called it, with only a few documented cases of yellow fever in their ranks. Other diseases—typhoid, malaria, and dysentery—however, took a far greater toll. In fact, the 2,500 disease fatalities suffered by American soldiers in Cuba outnumbered battlefield fatalities six to one. So once the brief American military effort ended, American officials launched a massive sanitation campaign. Streets in major cities and towns were cleaned daily by a legion of sweepers while water boys doused the swept streets with Electrozone—a sanitizing agent made from seawater. Even minor outbreaks triggered quarantines, while all luggage and goods shipped to the United States were disinfected, along with outgoing mail.[43]

Yet while extensive and elaborate, these sanitation efforts could not prevent the recurrence of yellow fever. Rooted as they were in miasmatic theories and ignorant of the mosquito's role in transmission, sanitation measures alone would never eradicate the disease. The more critical step taken by Surgeon General George Sternberg was his ordering of investigations into the primary infectious diseases threatening Cuba, especially yellow fever.[44]

Sternberg, America's leading authority on yellow fever, had spent more than twenty years trying to track down the microorganism that caused the disease. He had secured his place in bacteriological history by isolating the microorganism responsible for bacterial pneumonia in 1881. But in his pursuit of yellow fever's bacterial agent, he proved a better mythbuster than cure-finder—in Brazil, Mexico, and Cuba he disproved the conclusions of one researcher after another engaged in the same hunt. In 1897 he was particularly engaged in debunking the claim of Italian scientist Giuseppe Sanarelli that he had discovered the yellow fever bacterium. To help make the case, Sternberg ordered army physician Walter Reed to conduct research at the Army Medical College in Washington, D.C.[45]

Reed had studied medicine in his native state of Virginia before joining the army in 1875. Dispatched to Fort Yuma, Arizona, he spent almost two decades at a series of western appointments until called back to Washington by Sternberg to teach at the newly established army college. By the time he returned, medical science had been revolutionized. The bacterial organisms responsible for typhoid, tuberculosis, cholera, malaria, diphtheria, and tetanus had all been identified. Reed therefore jumped at the chance to join in these epidemiological investigations and enthusiastically accepted Sternberg's request to take charge of the yellow fever investigations in Cuba in 1900.[46]

When he began this research, Reed suspected that the disease was inhaled through the nose. Yet he was intrigued by Finlay's hypothesis, especially after the "guardhouse case" at Pinar del Rio. When a prisoner came down with yellow fever in a cell shared with eight others, it was assumed that some or all would soon contract the disease. When they did not, contagionist theories took a hit. To verify the resulting conclusion that the disease was not transferred through the contaminated bedding or clothing of the sick, Reed's team conducted human experiments. Three volunteers were confined nightly in a sealed barrack, sleeping on bedding soiled by yellow fever patients. When after three weeks of this regimen they did not contract the disease, the experiment was repeated with two other volunteers. When these also suffered no ill effects, Reed was convinced that lingering ideas about contagion and fomites had to be discarded altogether.[47]

Reed's team subsequently visited Finlay at his lab around 1 August and procured mosquito eggs for the study they had decided to conduct. Once

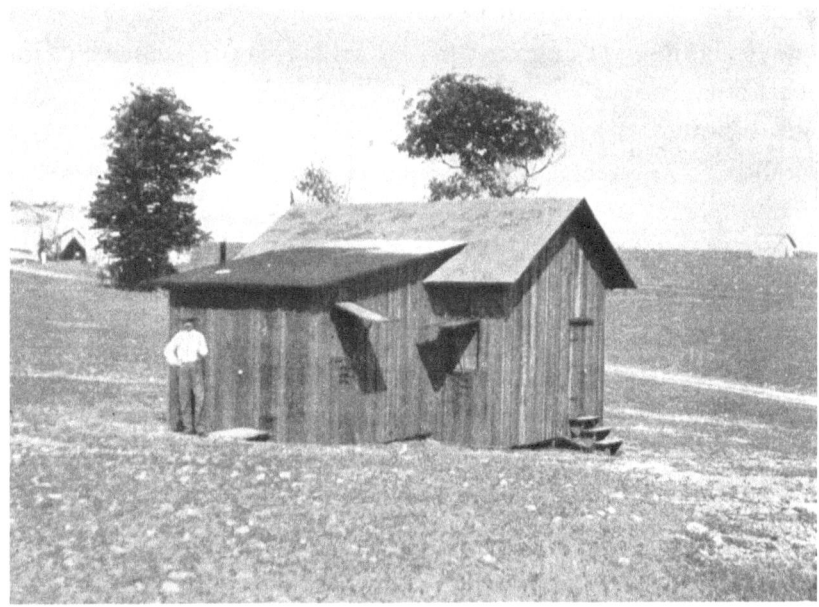

Walter Reed sealed volunteers in this hut to determine how yellow fever was transmitted. Photograph from *Walter Reed and Yellow Fever* by Howard A. Kelly, 1906. (Wellcome Collection)

hatched, mosquitoes were allowed to feed on yellow fever victims before being turned loose on the healthy arms of volunteers from the research team. The initial results were morbidly disappointing—none of the volunteers contracted the disease. But in late August, one of the volunteers, James Carroll, came down with fever. And on 25 September, Jesse Lazear, a physician who had left his position at Johns Hopkins Hospital to join the team, took sick and died.[48]

Reed was actually in the states at the time, but poring over Lazear's notebooks on his return to Cuba, he theorized the reasons behind the early "failures" and later tragically successful experiments. Henry Rose Carter, a field epidemiologist with the Marine Hospital Service, studying outbreaks in Mississippi had observed that the first case of yellow fever was often not followed by a second for another two weeks. Carter theorized that the infecting germ must undergo some sort of "extrinsic incubation" within an external, intermediate host between the time it left one victim and was transmitted to another. Applying this observation to the timeline laid out in Lazear's journals, Reed concluded that a mosquito, once ingesting the yellow fever microbe through biting a human carrier, incubated the microorganism for roughly fourteen days before being able to transfer the disease to another individual.[49]

It would be another twenty years for the yellow fever virus to be isolated, but with the vector/extrinsic incubator identified, the army was able to take rapid and amazingly effective steps to reduce mosquito populations. Rain barrels were covered, a sulfur-based fumigant was dispersed, and heavy oil was spread over ponds and other water sources suffocating the larvae before they could take flight. Within just a matter of months, yellow fever was all but eliminated in Cuba. Between September 1901 and July 1902, there were only two cases on the island.[50]

It is truly remarkable how dramatically Western understandings of disease changed over just a few decades at the end of the nineteenth century. Once Koch's work with anthrax was encapsulated within the postulates for identifying the causative microorganism behind several diseases, ancient ideas about humors and effluvia were largely abandoned. Nor is it possible to exaggerate Koch's direct influence on the American medical community. A handful of American physicians and researchers made the pilgrimage to Germany to work with the increasingly famous bacteriologist; the subsequent lines connecting Koch's work to Americans' success in unraveling the mysteries of yellow fever are easy to draw. For example, William Henry Welch, after being named professor of pathology at the newly established Johns Hopkins Medical School, traveled to Germany to study directly under Koch. George Sternberg was among Welch's first group of students at Johns Hopkins on Welch's return. Walter Reed did not study under Koch but he was joined in Cuba by Edward Shakespeare, who had studied briefly with Koch and then relied heavily on Koch's research in his own studies of cholera a decade before joining Reed.[51]

Germ theory's triumph was not complete. A few clung doggedly to the ancient but familiar concepts. Yet for the very great part, American physicians embraced the new theories and the therapies they recommended. The suddenness with which American medicine changed might be most simply attributed to the brilliance and effectiveness of the new science. Yet it could also be argued that American physicians were ready for something new. Traditional medical theories might have survived the great medical crises of the century but each challenge had done its part to chip away at confidence in these theories and the premises beneath them. The cholera epidemic left medical professionals skeptical about their ability to unravel the mysteries of disease, while the Civil War encouraged a batch of military physicians to rethink not just certain core tenets of their scientific educations but also the nature of medical research. If unable to put all the pieces together during the conflict, they had begun to recognize the greater complexity of disease and inch toward the conclusions European research made more evident.[52]

American doctors were not alone in clinging to ancient ideas for most of the nineteenth century—yet it is too simple and fundamentally unhistorical to dismiss the stagnation within American medicine as merely symptomatic within Western science more generally. Too much of the American story was shaped by a particular event in a particular city at a particular time.

In other words, the failures of American medicine, while certainly informed by broader failures, were shaped by factors peculiar to America—factors perhaps best illustrated by indulging in an intellectually suspect but provocative counterfactual exercise. What if this first epidemic had occurred in a different city, one not divided for decades into antagonistic camps? What if Philadelphia's yellow fever epidemic had prompted collegial research rather than intellectual warfare? What if Philadelphia's physicians had united in a search for best practices, or even more ambitiously, within a concentrated pursuit of the causative factors, research of the sort modeled by Isaac Cathrall in his study of black vomit? What if America's first, most prominent, and influential medical journal had been genuinely nonpartisan in its purposes, rather than the brainchild of a Rush disciple, a frustrated young intellectual seemingly more interested in carving out a distinctive place in American letters than orchestrating a balanced examination of health and disease?

Had America's medical leaders done a better job of reassuring an anxious public—had they been able to build public confidence rather than undermine it through public squabbles—would they have been able to maintain control over the diagnostic and therapeutic narrative rather than share the public forum with laypeople and quacks? And then later, would they have been better positioned to respond to the attacks of irregulars? Would they have been able to build more credible institutions, more respectable medical schools, rather than sacrifice the turf to proprietary, for-profit schools? Had the profession been more comfortably established, might it have been able to more effectively rebut or even learn from and absorb the useful and logical offered up by medical innovators rather than respond to them merely as threats to their power and authority? And perhaps most importantly, would all this have created a different intellectual climate—one more ambitious and receptive, one that might have turned rare but important breakthroughs like an understanding of puerperal fever into a broader understanding of infection, and one that would have had the courage to consider fringe theories like those of Josiah Nott even though they challenged central components of American ideology?

A different response in 1793 might have placed the medical profession's pursuit of public respect and diagnostic and therapeutic hegemony on better footing. It might have altered or accelerated the trajectory of the profession's advance, allowed it to more quickly earn recognition as "the authority" on matters related to health. But then, it might not have—or rather, it might have succeeded in these ways only if a more coherent and creative medical community was actually able to make real progress in its pursuit of medical answers. After all, given the rapidity with which germ theory revolutionized physicians' and lay understandings of disease, the medical community might have struggled to establish its intellectual authority until it developed more effective diagnostic tools and modes of therapy. In other words, in the end, the public's deferral to the voice of the medical establishment rested in large part on that establishment's ability to deliver better care and a more credible set of ideas.

If unable to do so, it would be logical that Americans would continue to place their own medical insights on par with those of their credentialed physicians, especially since so many of the older ideas to which they clung were so intricately woven into larger ideas within American culture about nature and knowledge. Miasmatic theories were supported by more comprehensive beliefs about the reliability of our senses and the benevolence of a god who purposely made the order of God's creation detectible by those senses. Heroic depletion therapies squared not just with the concomitant belief that the path to wellness could be measured by the demands any medicine or treatment imposed on the body but with the value Americans placed on self-mastery—the belief expressed in everything from conversion morphologies to republican ideology that health—religious, political, and physical—required discipline, self-denial, and the mastery of our weaker selves.

In the absence of paradigm-shifting discoveries about health and disease, rethinking inherited ideas would have required rethinking the larger constellation of ideas in which they were embedded. Yet still, it is worth pondering whether a different history, a different set of surrounding circumstances, might have made this sort of reconsideration more possible.

History is more appropriately the study of what is than what might have been. But the best history pays close attention to the particular as well as the general—the specific individuals, locations, and contexts in which events occur; the feuds that surround a new idea; the journals that host the discussion; and even the personalities of those at the center. It pays attention to the particularity within any event and is suspicious of the suggestion that any path is inevitable. For almost a century, American disease theory advanced little. While other fields of science made significant strides, America's doctors clung to two-thousand-year-old etiologies and employed centuries-old therapeutics. A series of what-ifs does not necessarily mean that an alternative was possible, but the particulars within this history should remind us that the story of American medicine in the nineteenth century was not etched in stone.

NOTES

Introduction

1. Funk, "Key Findings about Americans' Confidence in Science"; Funk, Kennedy, and Johnson, "Trust in Medical Scientists Has Grown." This overwhelming support for vaccination programs belies the resistance federal initiatives faced during the 1950s and 1960s; see Conis, *Vaccine Nation*.
2. Funk, "Polling Shows Signs of Public Trust in Institutions."
3. On the practice of medicine in early America, see Abrams, *Revolutionary Medicine*; Burnham, *Health Care in America*; Bell, *The Colonial Physician*; Murphy, *Enter the Physician*; Breslaw, *Lotions, Potions, Pills, and Magic*; Rothstein, *American Physicians in the Nineteenth Century*; and Rutkow, *Seeking the Cure*. See also Bell, *John Morgan*.
4. For a wide-ranging exploration of humoral medicine from antiquity to the present, see Arikha, *Passions and Tempers*.
5. On the role of depletion therapies in early American medicine, see Sullivan, "Sanguine Practices"; Estes, "Therapeutic Practice in Colonial New England"; Warner, *The Therapeutic Perspective*; and Duffy, *From Humors to Medical Science*.
6. See Rosenberg, "The Therapeutic Revolution."
7. Child mortality rates are particularly striking. Infant mortality may have been as high as 40 percent in the last decades of the eighteenth century; in Philadelphia during the 1780s, children under ten accounted for roughly half of all deaths. Abrams, *Revolutionary Medicine*, 13.
8. In tracking this public debate this study draws heavily from Andrew Brown's Philadelphia *Federal Gazette*. The city's other major dailies—the *Pennsylvania Packet*, the *Gazette of the United States*, the *General Advertiser*, and *The Mail or Claypoole's Daily Advertiser*—suspended publication during the epidemic.
9. Bartlett quoted in Shryock, "The Fielding H. Garrison Lecture," 525.
10. See Carr, *The Topography of Wellness*, 22–23; Devine, *Learning from the Wounded*, 6; King, *Transformations in American Medicine*, 1–18; and Duffy, *The Healers*, 98.

11. Quoted in Peterson, *Thomas Jefferson and the New Nation*, 253; Thomas Jefferson to William Green Mumford, June 18, 1799, in Koch, ed., *The American Enlightenment*, 340.
12. Rush, "Observations on the Duties of a Physician," 455; Rush, "An Inquiry into the Natural History of Medicine," 114.
13. Rush, "Observations on the Duties of a Physician," 455–56.
14. Powell, *Bring Out Your Dead*, 179, 175; Griffith, "'A Total Dissolution of the Bonds of Society,'" 56.
15. McMahon, "Beyond Therapeutics," 112, 114; Nord, "Readership as Citizenship," 21, 36.
16. Lapsansky, "'Abigail, a Negress,'" 69, 61; Allen and Jones, *A Narrative*, 13.
17. Bliss, *The Making of Modern Medicine*, 7–30.

1. 1793

1. The most useful account of the epidemic's early weeks remains Powell, *Bring Out Your Dead*. Mathew Carey provided a contemporary account in *A Short Account of the Malignant Fever*. There is evidence that the disease originated in West Africa and that Haitian refugees were infected after signing on ships traveling from that continent—or perhaps acquired the disease not in Saint-Domingue but rather while passing through other British colonies receiving ships from West Africa. See Smith, *Ship of Death*, and Blake, "Yellow Fever in Eighteenth-Century America."
2. Mortality statistics were recorded in Hardie, *An Account of the Rise, Progress, and Termination of the Malignant Fever*. Rush published his recommendations for the first time in the *Federal Gazette* on September 12. He summarized the evolution of his analysis and discovery of a treatment in *An Account of the Bilious Remitting Yellow Fever*.
3. See Powell, *Bring Out Your Dead*, 140–94.
4. Ibid., 95–101. On the response of the Black community to Benjamin Rush's plea that they serve as caregivers during the crisis, see Allen and Jones, *A Narrative*, and Will, "Liberalism, Republicanism, and Philadelphia's Black Elite."
5. Drinker, *The Diary of Elizabeth Drinker*.
6. Burial numbers are from Hardie, *An Account of the Rise, Progress, and Termination of the Malignant Fever*.
7. Susan E. Klepp offers a more detailed look at mortality rates during the epidemic in "'How Many Precious Souls Are Fled.'"
8. McNeill, *Mosquito Empires*, 16; Crosby, "Virgin Soil Epidemics." Suzanne Austin Alchon provides a detailed review of the epidemics striking the Americas after European contact in *A Pest in the Land*.
9. Grob, *The Deadly Truth*, 15–25.
10. Alchon, *A Pest in the Land*.
11. For the following paragraphs, see McNeill, *Mosquito Empires*, especially 15–188.
12. For more than you might ever want to know about mosquitoes, see Richard Jones's *Mosquito*.

13. In addition to McNeill, see Bewell, *Romanticism and Colonial Disease*, on the British interest in "medical geography."
14. Quoted in Hogarth, *Medicalizing Blackness*, 22.
15. Ibid. In addition to Hogarth, see Espinosa, "The Question of Racial Immunity."
16. Johnston, *The Nature of Slavery*.
17. Savitt, *Medicine and Slavery*, 241; Humphreys, *Yellow Fever and the South*, 7. For a more complete introduction to this position, see Carrigan, "Privilege, Prejudice, and the Strangers' Disease," and Kiple and Kiple, "Black Yellow Fever Immunities."
18. Hogarth, *Medicalizing Blackness*, 30; McNeill, *Mosquito Empires*, 45.
19. Yellow fever remains a threat on three continents, with the World Health Organization estimating as many as 200,000 cases and 30,000–60,000 fatalities annually. While massive vaccination campaigns in West Africa have reduced the risk of epidemics there, eastern and central African countries remain at far greater risk. More than a dozen countries in Latin America are susceptible to yellow fever epidemics, as well as Asian countries like China and India, with large populations with no historical contact and thus immunities, as well as large populations of the specific *Aedes aegypti* mosquito vector. These facts inspired the World Health Organization to launch a new vaccination campaign in 2017. See *A Global Strategy to Eliminate Yellow Fever*.

2. Benjamin Rush Gives an Ancient Theory a New Twist

1. Over the next several decades, even as ideas about yellow fever evolved, coffee remained an especially suspicious item. Cargos were routinely quarantined and even turned back by officials manning the quarantine station outside Philadelphia; see Barnes, "Cargo, 'Infection,' and the Logic of Quarantine," and Barnes, *Lazaretto*.
2. *Federal Gazette*, Aug. 28, 1793. On the miasmatic theories widely embraced in early America, see Valenčius, *The Health of the Country*, especially 109–32.
3. Rush, *An Account of the Bilious Remitting Yellow Fever*, 167. On the mortality rate during the epidemic, see Klepp, "'How Many Precious Souls Are Fled?'"
4. On Rush's life, see Brodsky, *Benjamin Rush*; D'Elia, *Benjamin Rush*; and Eric T. Carlson, Jeffrey L. Wollock, and Patrick S. Noel, introduction, in Rush, *Benjamin Rush's Lectures on the Mind*, 1–44. See also Unger, *Dr. Benjamin Rush*; Fried, *Rush*; and Naramore, *Benjamin Rush*.
5. Rush's views on slavery were contained in *An Address to the Inhabitants of the British Settlements in America upon Slave Keeping*. Rush described the mixed reception he received in Philadelphia as well as his controversy-filled military experience in his autobiography, *The Autobiography of Benjamin Rush*, 78–89, 131–37.
6. Seventy-two students enrolled in the Institutes of Medicine when Rush first taught the course in 1791; in 1810, 369 students enrolled. It is estimated that Rush taught more than 3,000 students during his career from 1779–1813. Rush, *Benjamin Rush's Lectures on the Mind*, 16–17.

7. Ibid., 85. John Brown's *Elements of Medicine* was first published in 1780 and translated into English in 1788. He, like Rush, had studied under William Cullen at Edinburgh, perhaps explaining why Rush, even while quoting Brown, was anxious to trace the broader concept to views formerly taught by their mentor. Cullen later abandoned this view of the body, but when Rush took his course in 1771, Cullen taught that "the human body is not an automaton or self-moving machine, but is kept alive and in motion by the constant action of stimuli upon it." Rush, *Benjamin Rush's Lectures on the Mind*, 86.
8. Ibid., 94, 99.
9. Ibid., 100.
10. Rush, *Benjamin Rush's Lectures on the Mind*, 87, 103, 186. On the relation between the moral sense and sensory stimulus see Carlson and Simpson, "Benjamin Rush's Medical Use of the Moral Faculty."
11. Rush, *Benjamin Rush's Lectures on the Mind*, 104, 109–10, 113.
12. Rush's shift in terminology reflected his growing dependence on John Brown. Francis Glisson had first suggested that the body was laced with some sort of reflexive substance in the seventeenth century and labeled it "irritability." Albrecht von Haller took this theory a step further, labeling the muscular substance that reacted to coarse stimuli, producing movement, "irritability," and tissue that reacted to more subtle stimuli, producing thought and emotion, "sensibility." In his earliest lectures Rush used von Haller's terms, and he never fully abandoned Haller's dual taxonomy, but he increasingly incorporated Brown's ideas and labels. Brown argued that the key to life was the ability "to be affected by external agents" and renamed Haller's irritability and sensibility "excitability," and the lifeforce or energy produced when a stimulant interacted with excitability "excitement." See Rush, *Benjamin Rush's Lectures on the Mind*, in particular 54–56, 231–34.
13. Ibid., 131–32, 137–39.
14. Ibid., 129.
15. Ibid., 117.
16. Brown, *The Elements of Medicine*, 14, 137.
17. Rush, *Benjamin Rush's Lectures on the Mind*, 188, 190–91. See also Brown, *The Elements of Medicine*, especially 290–312.
18. Rush, *An Account of the Bilious Remitting Yellow Fever*, 12.
19. Ibid., 28, 104.
20. Ibid., 30, 35. Rush's terminology can be misleading—he used terms like "toxin" and "contagion" without intending (or understanding) the words in their modern sense. The debate that developed over the origins and nature of the disease would force Rush and other disputants to sharpen their language.
21. Ibid., 31–33, 100.
22. *Federal Gazette*, Sept. 16, 1793.
23. Rush, *An Account of the Bilious Remitting Yellow Fever*, 193–95.
24. Benjamin Rush to Julia Rush, Aug. 25, 1793, in Rush, *Letters of Benjamin Rush*, 2:640–43.

25. Rush, "An Inquiry into the Natural History of Medicine," 136–39; Benjamin Rush to Julia Rush, Aug. 25, 1793, in Rush, *Letters of Benjamin Rush*, 2:640–43.
26. Benjamin Rush to Elizabeth Graeme Fergusson, Jan. 18, 1793; Benjamin Rush to Julia Rush, Aug. 21, 29, 1793, in ibid., 2:627–29, 637–39, 644–45, 646–47.
27. Mitchell quoted in Rush, *An Account of the Bilious Remitting Yellow Fever*, 198.
28. Benjamin Rush to Julia Rush, Sept. 5, 1793, in Rush, *Letters of Benjamin Rush*, 2:650–52.
29. Rush, *An Account of the Bilious Remitting Yellow Fever*, 204; Benjamin Rush to Julia Rush, Sept. 18, 1793, in Rush, *Letters of Benjamin Rush*, 2:668–71. See also *Federal Gazette*, Sept. 12, Oct. 7, 1793.
30. Bartlett quoted in Shryock, "The Fielding H. Garrison Lecture," 525; Powell, *Bring Out Your Dead*, 122, 129.
31. Kopperman, "'Venerate the Lancet,'" 567.
32. Bailyn, *Ideological Origins of the American Revolution*; Apel, *Feverish Bodies, Enlightened Minds*, 136.
33. Holmes, "Benjamin Rush and the Yellow Fever."
34. Rush, *An Account of the Bilious Remitting Yellow Fever*, 247, also 244–74.
35. Rush, *Benjamin Rush's Lectures on the Mind*, 238–44.
36. Rush, *An Account of the Bilious Remitting Yellow Fever*, 245–46.
37. On the relationship between Rush's views and those of contemporaries, see Kopperman, "'Venerate the Lancet.'" For regional practices, see Waring, "The Influence of Benjamin Rush on the Practice of Bleeding."
38. Rush summarized (and addressed) these criticisms in *An Account of the Bilious Remitting Yellow Fever*, 249–55, 274–77.
39. Kuhn presented his therapeutic recommendation in the *Federal Gazette* for the first time on 11 September. His ally Dr. Edward Stevens offered his recommendations in the *Gazette* on 16 September. Rush, "Lecture upon the Causes Which Have Retarded the Progress of Medicine," 143; Rush, *An Account of the Bilious Remitting Yellow Fever*, 258; Benjamin Rush to Julia Rush, Sept. 23, 1793, in Rush, *Letters of Benjamin Rush*, 2:676–78.
40. *Federal Gazette*, Sept. 12, 14, 23, 1793. See also Benjamin Rush, "An Account of the Origins, Symptoms, and Treatment of the Epidemic Fever," *Federal Gazette*, Oct. 7, 1793.
41. Ramsey, *An Eulogium upon Benjamin Rush*, 23; Powell, *Bring Out Your Dead*, 127; D'Elia, "Dr. Benjamin Rush and the American Medical Revolution."
42. On Rush's persisting influence, despite the criticism of some contemporaries, see Shryock, "The Fielding H. Garrison Lecture."

3. Philadelphia's Medical Establishment

1. *The Charter, Constitution, and By Laws of the College of Physicians*; Olton, "Philadelphia's First Environmental Class." See also McMahon, "Beyond Therapeutics," and Finger, *The Contagious City*. On the motivations of hospital founders, see Williams, "The

'Industrious Poor' and the Founding of the Pennsylvania Hospital." Ben Mutschler offers a deeper look at the ways in which early American communities tended to their sick in *The Province of Affliction*.
2. *The Charter, Constitution, and By Laws of the College of Physicians*.
3. See Corner, *Shippen*, and Bell, *John Morgan*.
4. Bard's letter is reprinted in Corner, *Shippen*, 95; Ruston's is excerpted in Bell, *John Morgan*, 112.
5. Rosner, "Thistle on the Delaware."
6. Corner, *Shippen*, 50–95; Louis, "William Shippen's Unsuccessful Attempt to Establish the First 'School for Physick.'"
7. Louis, "William Shippen's Unsuccessful Attempt to Establish the First 'School for Physick,'" 226–27, 233–37.
8. Bell, *John Morgan*, 76–99. On Shippen's obstetrics practice, see Leavitt, "'Science' Enters the Birthing Room."
9. Bell, *John Morgan*, 100–128; Corner, *Shippen*, 111.
10. Bell, *John Morgan*, 44–75; Morgan, *A Discourse upon the Institution of Medical Schools in America*. While Shippen was a very good student, it is hard to find evidence of intellectual curiosity in his record. The brief diary he kept while studying in London records little more than his daily activities, and his robust social life receives as much attention as his class schedule. There is no comment on the substance of his studies, no hint of enthusiasm or fascination. Nor did Shippen compile a professional resume that might suggest an interest in the medical, scientific, or even political questions of his time. He published nothing, conducted no research, and left only a few letters. Upon his death, Benjamin Rush called Shippen "indolent." Even his sympathetic biographer concedes he was "uncontemplative."
11. Morgan, *A Discourse upon the Institution of Medical Schools in America*, 34–35; Corner, *Shippen*, 109–10.
12. Thomas Bond to Benjamin Franklin, June 7, 1769, Founders Online, National Archives, https://founders.archives.gov/documents/Franklin/01-16-02-0075.
13. See Corner, *Shippen*, 180.
14. Bell, *John Morgan*, 178–205.
15. Ibid.
16. Ibid.
17. Ibid., 206–39; Morgan, *A Vindication of His Public Character*, xxiv; Morgan, *To the Citizens and Freemen of the United States of America*.
18. Quoted in Bell, *John Morgan*, 219.
19. For Rush's childhood and education, see Brodsky, *Benjamin Rush*, and Carlson, Wollock, and Noel's introduction to Rush, *Benjamin Rush's Lectures on the Mind*, 1–44.
20. Benjamin Rush to John Adams, Oct. 1, 21, 1777; Rush to Nathanael Greene, Dec. 2, 1777; Rush to William Duer, Dec. 8, 13, 1777; Rush to George Washington, Dec. 26, 1777, in Rush, *Letters of Benjamin Rush*, 1:154–57, 159–63, 168–69, 171–77, 180–82.
21. Benjamin Rush to John Adams, Oct. 21, 1777, in ibid., 1:159–63.

22. Benjamin Rush to William Duer, Dec. 8, 1777, in ibid., 1:171–74. Rush later described his appearance before Congress in a letter to John Morgan in June (?) 1779, in ibid., 1:225–29.
23. Rush to George Washington, Feb. 25, 1778; Rush to Nathanael Greene, Feb. 1, 1778; Rush to Daniel Roberdeau, March 9, 1778, in ibid., 1:200–204, 194–96, 204–8.
24. Benjamin Rush to John Morgan, June 1779, quoted in Corner, *Shippen*, 225.
25. Bell, *John Morgan*, 220–40; Bell, "The Court Martial of William Shippen, Jr."
26. "Depositions" and "Dr. Morgan's Continuation," *Pennsylvania Packet*, Sept. 9; Oct. 7, 21, 28; Nov. 4, 11; Dec. 23, 1780.
27. "Dr. Morgan's Appeal to the Free Citizens of the United States of America," *Pennsylvania Packet*, Sept. 2, 1780; "Dr. Morgan's Continuation," *Pennsylvania Packet*, Oct. 14, 1780.
28. William Shippen, "To the Public," *Pennsylvania Packet*, Nov. 11, 1780; "Dr. Shippen's Vindication," *Pennsylvania Packet*, Nov. 18, 25; Dec. 6, 1780.
29. Benjamin Rush, "To Dr. William Shippen, Jr.," *Pennsylvania Packet*, Nov. 21, 1780; Rush deposition excerpted in "Dr. Morgan's Continuation," *Pennsylvania Packet*, Oct. 7, 1780.
30. James Hutchinson deposition excerpted in "Dr. Morgan's Continuation," *Pennsylvania Packet*, Oct. 7, 1780.
31. Benjamin Rush, "To Dr. William Shippen, Jr.," *Pennsylvania Packet*, Dec. 2, 1780; "Letter from Thomas Bond, Jr.," *Pennsylvania Packet*, Dec. 9, 1780.
32. Morgan, "To William Shippen, Jr., Esq.," *Pennsylvania Packet*, Dec. 23, 1780.
33. Calamus (Francis Hopkinson), "For the Pennsylvania Packet," *Pennsylvania Packet*, Dec. 23, 1780.
34. Morgan, *Doctor Morgan's Remarks on Dr. Shippen's Feeble Attempts*.
35. Although all were eventually named to the faculty after a contentious dispute, Morgan never assumed his teaching duties.
36. Useful introductions to the evolution of American medicine and medical practice during the late colonial and early national periods include Burnham, *Health Care in America*; Numbers, ed., *The Education of American Physicians*; Ludmerer, *Learning to Heal*; Rothstein, *American Physicians in the Nineteenth Century*; Starr, *The Transformation of American Medicine*; and Murphy, *Enter the Physician*.
37. Porter, "Before the Fringe," 3.
38. See Fenn, *Pox Americana*, 31–42. Americans bristled at Sutton's claim that his methods were innovative; they argued that during the 1730s American inoculators introduced the use of lymph from an inoculee rather than a natural victim, and Sutton's supposedly innovative preparatory regimen included the same mercury compounds utilized by Americans. In addition to Fenn, see Wehrman, *The Contagion of Liberty*, 129–35. Using infectious material drawn from a natural smallpox victim, fatality rates due to inoculation were as high as 10 percent.
39. Fenn, *Pox Americana*. See also Abrams, *Revolutionary Medicine*, 132–41.
40. Fenn, *Pox Americana*; Dine, "Diaries and Doctors"; Wehrman, "The Siege of 'Castle Pox.'"

41. Adams quoted in Wehrman, *The Contagion of Liberty*, 122.
42. Fenn, *Pox Americana*, 38–40; Dine, "Diaries and Doctors," 420.
43. Fenn, *Pox Americana*, 33–35; Dine, "Diaries and Doctors." Rush described the particulars of his inoculation process in *The New Method of Inoculating for the Smallpox*. See also Gronim, "Imagining Inoculation."
44. Porter and Porter, "The Rise of the English Drug Industry"; Porter, "Before the Fringe," 10; Porter, "The Patient in England," 104.
45. Cook and Walker, "Circulation of Medicine in the Early Modern Atlantic World"; Wilson, "Trading in Drugs through Philadelphia." See also Griffenhagen and Young, "Old English Patent Medicines."
46. Lawrence, "William Buchan."
47. The discussion here and below is based on a sampling of the following Philadelphia newspapers between 1767 and 1793: the *Pennsylvania Chronicle*, *Pennsylvania Packet*, *Pennsylvania Evening Post*, *Pennsylvania Federal Gazette*, and *Dunlap's American Daily Advertiser*.
48. Morgan, *A Discourse upon the Institution of Medical Schools in America*; Cowen, "Colonial Laws Pertaining to Pharmacy"; Wilson, and Savacool, "The Theory and Practice of Pharmacy in Pennsylvania."
49. See note 47 for the newspapers reviewed for this discussion. Specific references to Yardell and Weed can be found in *Pennsylvania Evening Post*, March 18, Aug. 26, Oct. 14, 1777.
50. Loudin, "The Vile Race of Quacks."
51. Edward Hazen suggested that druggists, chemists, apothecaries, and physicians had managed to carve out distinct spheres of operation by midcentury in "The Druggist and the Apothecary," first published in 1841.
52. Morgan, *A Discourse upon the Institution of Medical Schools in America*; Gelfand, "The Origins of a Modern Concept of Medical Specialization."
53. Rush, "Observations on the Duties of a Physician," 437.
54. Rush, "On the Means of Acquiring Business"; Rush, "On the Duties of Patients to Their Physicians."
55. Rosner, "Thistle on the Delaware."
56. Bell, *The College of Physicians*. See also Bell, *John Morgan*, 136–40.
57. *The Charter, Constitution, and By Laws of the College of Physicians*. See also Bell, *The College of Physicians*, 1–25.
58. Bell, *The College of Physicians*, 18–19.
59. Ibid., 19–20.

4. The Fractured Response to the 1793 Epidemic

1. "College of Physicians' Report," *Federal Gazette*, Aug. 27, 1793.
2. *Federal Gazette*, Aug. 28, 27, 31, 29, 1793; Powell, *Bring Out Your Dead*, 23–24.

3. *Dunlap's American Daily Advertiser*, Aug. 29, 1793. This was not the first time the significance of an unusually large mosquito population went unrecognized. During a 1780 outbreak of "break-bone fever"—probably dengue fever—Benjamin Rush offered the abundant mosquitoes as evidence of an "unwholesome atmosphere," in other words, proof of his miasmatic theories rather than the vector they actually were. Quoted in Packard, "'Break-Bone' Fever," 195.
4. Currie, *A Description of the Malignant, Infectious Fever*, 6.
5. *Federal Gazette*, Sept. 11, 1793.
6. Ibid., Sept. 12, 13, 1793.
7. Ibid., Sept. 13, 17, 1793.
8. Ibid., Sept. 14, 1793.
9. Ibid., Sept. 18, 19, 17, 23, 14, 1793.
10. Ibid., Sept. 24, 1793.
11. Ibid., Sept. 27, 1793.
12. Ibid., Sept. 20, 1793. See also Smith, "Andrew Brown's 'Earnest Endeavor.'"
13. Deveze, *An Enquiry into and Observations*, 16, 34.
14. Ibid., 47–48.
15. Nassy, *Observations on the Cause, Nature, and Treatment of the Epidemic Disorder*, 43.
16. Ibid., 39.
17. Pascalis-Ouvière, *An Account of the Contagious Epidemic Yellow Fever*, 23. See also Middleton, "Felix Pascalis-Ouvière."
18. Currie, *A Dissertation on the Autumnal Remitting Fever*, 7.
19. Hardie, *An Account of the Rise, Progress, and Termination of the Malignant Fever*.
20. Chisholm, *An Essay on the Malignant Pestilential Fever*, 83; Smith, *Ship of Death*.
21. Smith, *Ship of Death*, 157–86.
22. Currie, *A Description of the Malignant, Infectious Fever*, 6, 14.
23. Powell, *Bring Out Your Dead*, 84; Currie, *A Description of the Malignant, Infectious Fever*, 14.
24. Currie, *An Historical Account of the Climate*.
25. Ibid., 110, 95, 192.
26. Currie, *Of the Cholera*, 2.
27. Cathrall, *A Medical Sketch of the Synochus Maligna*, 10–12; Currie and Cathrall, *Facts and Observations*.
28. Cathrall, *Memoir on the Analysis of the Black Vomit*, 21, 23.
29. Ffirth, *A Treatise on Malignant Fever*.
30. Benjamin Rush to Philadelphia Committee of Health, Sept. 13, 1794; Rush to John Redman Coxe, Sept. 19, 1794, in Rush, *Letters of Benjamin Rush*, 2:749–50, 750–51.
31. For news of the New Haven and Baltimore outbreaks, see *Philadelphia Gazette and Universal Daily Advertiser*, Aug. 20, 1794, and *Gazette of the United States*, Sept. 1, 1794. Mifflin's proclamation first appeared in the *Philadelphia Gazette and Universal Daily Advertiser*, Aug. 22, 1794. New York's suspension of trade was reported in the

Philadelphia Gazette and Universal Daily Advertiser, Sept. 2, 1794. The Baltimore health committee's denial of "Yellow Fever or other contagious disease" was reported in the *Philadelphia Gazette and Universal Daily Advertiser*, Aug. 30, 1794. The suspension of trade between Baltimore and Philadelphia was reported in the *Philadelphia Gazette and Universal Daily Advertiser*, Oct. 6, 1794.

32. *Philadelphia Gazette*, Oct. 4, 1794.
33. *The Argus, or Greenleaf's New Daily Advertiser*, Aug. 12, 14, 17, 26; Sept. 4, 5, 1795; *Philadelphia Gazette*, Sept. 24, 1795.
34. *Philadelphia Gazette*, Sept. 24, 1795.
35. *Porcupine's Gazette*, Sept. 18, 1797; *Gazette of the United States*, Sept. 18, 1797.
36. *Porcupine's Gazette*, Sept. 19, 1797; *Gazette of the United States*, Sept. 18, 19, 1797.
37. *Gazette of the United States*, Oct. 3, 1797.
38. Ibid., Oct. 5, 1797.
39. Ibid., Oct. 6, 1797.
40. The exchange between Currie and Wynkoop was published in the *Gazette of the United States*, Oct. 10–12, Nov. 2–3, 1797. Coxe's defense of Rush was contained in letters printed in the same paper, Oct. 16; Nov. 6, 9, 10, 14, 1797. Allen and Jones issued their own defense of the African American community's response to the crisis in *A Narrative*. They pointed out that while their Black neighbors embraced Rush's invitation to provide care for the sick, and even bled as many as eight hundred victims, their critic, Mathew Carey, fled the city in the early weeks of the epidemic. Carey's criticism was contained in *A Short Account of the Malignant Fever*.
41. *Gazette of the United States*, Nov. 6, 9, 10, 14, 1797.
42. *Porcupine's Gazette*, Oct. 3, 1797.
43. See, for example, ibid., Sept. 22, 28, 1797.
44. *Gazette of the United States*, Aug. 22, 1798.
45. Ibid., Sept. 13, 1798.
46. Ibid., Sept. 3, 1798.

5. America's First Medical Journals and the Battle for Authority

1. Waterman, *Republic of Intellect*, 3; May, *The Enlightenment in America*, 233.
2. Not all historians agree with this assessment of the *Repository*. Eve Kornfield suggests it answered the "clarion call" to medical and scientific advancement in the wake of the epidemic. Kornfield, "Crisis in the Capital."
3. A short biography of Smith is found in Smith, *The Diary of Elihu Hubbard Smith*.
4. Ibid., 43, 58–59, 80.
5. Ibid., 95, 99, 183.
6. Webster, *A Collection of Papers on the Subject of Bilious Fevers*.
7. On Webster's decision, see Elihu Hubbard Smith to William Buel, Aug. 11, 1796, in Smith, *The Diary of Elihu Hubbard Smith*, 201. On Smith's sense of inadequacy, see the

prefaces to his June and July 1796 entries, in Smith, *The Diary of Elihu Hubbard Smith*, 173, 183. Although deciding to not publish a second collection of letters, Webster did return to his study of disease. He submitted twenty-five letters to the *Commercial Advertiser* on the topic in late 1797, and in 1799 he published *A Brief History of Epidemic and Pestilential Diseases*.

8. Circular Letter to Physicians, Aug. 17, 1796, in Smith, *The Diary of Elihu Hubbard Smith*, 202; Elihu Hubbard Smith, "Letters to William Buel," in Webster, *A Collection of Papers on the Subject of Bilious Fevers*, 104; Elihu Hubbard Smith to Benjamin Rush, Sept. 9, 1796, in Smith, *The Diary of Elihu Hubbard Smith*, 214–17.
9. Elihu Hubbard Smith to Benjamin Rush, Sept. 9, 1796, in Smith, *The Diary of Elihu Hubbard Smith*, 217, 221.
10. Smith, "The Plague of Athens," 32. Thomas Apel discusses the philosophical and methodological bases of these sorts of historically based theories of disease in "The Thucydidean Moment."
11. "Review of *Medical Inquiries and Observations*," no. 1, 79; "Dr. Morton's Summary," 57; "Observations upon the Yellow Fever," 169.
12. "Review of *An Inaugural Essay*," 229–31; "Letter from the College of Physicians to Governor Mifflin"; Rush, "Letter of Dr. Rush and Others to Governor Mifflin"; "Review of *Medical Inquiries and Observations*," no. 3, 342.
13. Brown, "An Account of the Pestilential Disease Which Prevailed at Boston"; Channing, "An Account of the Pestilential Disease at New London"; Browne, "Treatise on the Yellow Fever"; "Review of *Memoirs of the Yellow Fever* by William Currie."
14. Wheaton, "A Brief Account of the Yellow Fever."
15. Beguerie, "Histoire de la fievre." See also Alibert, "A Treatise on Malignant Intermittents." The international dimensions of this debate are explored in Katherine Arner, "Making Yellow Fever American."
16. "Observations on the Preceding Paper"; Currie, "Notice of the Yellow Fever."
17. Shattuck, "An Essay on the Influence of Air upon Animal Bodies," 4.
18. Smith, "Facts and Observations Relative to the Bilious Remitting Fever," 19–22; "Facts and Observations, Chiefly Relative to the Yellow Fever."
19. "Medical Extracts," 71.
20. "Letter from Doctor James Mann on the Treatment of Croup"; Danielson and Mann, "The History of a Singular and Very Mortal Disease," 67.
21. "Observations on Certain Cases of Secondary Disease, Subsequent to the Measles"; "An Account of Two Cases of Dropsy," 402; Mease, "Account of the Efficacy of the External Application of the Geranium Maculatum"; "An Account of the Efficacy of Salivation in Curing Pulmonary Consumption," 400.
22. "An Account of the Good Effects of Copious Blood Letting in the Cure of a Hemorrhage," 1, 2.
23. Ibid., 5.
24. "Extract from the Asiatic Annual Register," 234.
25. See Hogarth, *Medicalizing Blackness*, 104–30, and Savitt, *Medicine and Slavery*, 171–84.

26. Dewees, "On the Efficacy of Blood-Letting," 27, 29. See also "An Account of the Effects of Copious Blood-Letting," 174–75.
27. Watkins, "On the Utility of Spirit of Turpentine in a Severe Burn"; Dewees, "An Attempt to Explain Why More Children Live," 280.
28. Elmer, "Case of Mortification and Separation of the Body of the Uterus"; "Fetus Found in the Abdomen of a Boy"; Clark, "Case of Extra-Uterine Gestation"; "Case of Superfoetation."
29. Vaughan, "Account of Two Albinos," 284.
30. Goldson, *Cases of Small Pox, Subsequent to Vaccination*.
31. For an introduction to Jenner and his work, see Smith, *The Man Who Saved the World from Smallpox*. See also Rusnock, "Catching Cowpox."
32. The term "vaccination"—derived from the Spanish word for cow, *vaca*—was first used to differentiate Jenner's treatment from the more traditional forms of inoculation in 1803. Until 1891, it was used in reference to smallpox only. But in that year, Louis Pasteur proposed its use for all prophylactic therapies to honor Jenner.
33. Mark and Rigan-Pérez, "The World's First Immunization Campaign"; Bowers, "The Odyssey of Smallpox Vaccination."
34. Gehlbach, *American Plagues*, 41–58.
35. On Jefferson's vaccination project, see Savitt, *Medicine and Slavery*, 293–97.
36. The following paragraphs rely heavily on Wehrman, *Contagion of Liberty*, especially 156–218, 282–318.
37. Goldson, *Cases of Small Pox, Subsequent to Vaccination*; "Medical Register"; Church, "Observations on Mr. Goldson's Pamphlet," 323; "Observations on Vaccination," 434. See also Rousseau, "More Proof of Vaccination's Effectiveness."
38. "Medical and Philosophical Register," 1, no. 2, 224–25; "An Account of the Introduction of the Vaccine Disease."
39. "Medical and Philosophical Register," 1, no. 3; "Vaccine Inoculation," 455.
40. "Dr. John Spence to the Editor," 401.
41. "Harris," "History of a Fatal Case of Hydrocephalus," 396; Dewees, "Case of a Ruptured Uterus."
42. Powell, *Bring Out Your Dead*, 123; Benjamin Rush to Elias Boudinot, Sept. 25, 1793, in Rush, *Letters of Benjamin Rush*, 2:680–82. See also Benjamin Rush to Julia Rush, Sept. 18, 1793, in Rush, *Letters of Benjamin Rush*, 2:668–71, and Rush, *An Account of the Bilious Remitting Yellow Fever*, 253.
43. Ackerknecht, "Anticontagionism."
44. Blake, "Yellow Fever in Eighteenth-Century America."
45. Valenčius, *The Health of the Country*, 122–23. For a more thorough discussion of the role of "smell" in locating threats to public health, see Kiechle, *Smell Detectives*.
46. Adam Kuhn and William Currie both argued that most victims suffered from only common bilious fevers. Kuhn claimed that between 23 August and 3 September he treated sixty patients and only seven actually had yellow fever. *Federal Gazette*, Sept. 13, 1793. Currie mocked Rush more directly: "Have we all got the yellow fever in

our bodies, only waiting for some exciting cause to put it into action? By no means. The disease which Dr. Rush calls the yellow fever . . . is only the fall fever." *Federal Gazette,* Sept. 17, 1793.

47. Stearns, *An Account of the Terrible Effects of the Pestilential Infection,* 1–2.
48. See Nassy, *Observations on the Cause, Nature, and Treatment of the Epidemic Disorder;* Deveze, *An Inquiry into and Observations;* Cathrall, *A Medical Sketch of the Synochus Maligna;* and Currie, *A Description of the Malignant, Infectious Fever.*
49. Rush, *An Account of the Bilious Remitting Yellow Fever,* 256; *Federal Gazette,* Oct. 1, Sept. 18, Oct. 3, 21, 1793. There is a similar celebration of heroic endurance in the letters from a Dr. Drysdale to his former teacher Rush while describing the yellow fever outbreak in Baltimore in 1784. One patient boasted that he "did not sink" under the operation of the purge that produced forty stools. Another claimed that he was cured by the purge-and-bleed treatment but it felt like needles darting through his body. "Dr. Drysdale's History of the Yellow Fever."
50. See Rosenberg, "The Therapeutic Revolution." J. Worth Estes has similarly suggested that the foul taste, the bitterness within patent medicines, was part of their appeal. In fact, he argues, "attitudes equating bad taste with efficacy" persisted well beyond the nineteenth century. Estes, "The Pharmacology of Nineteenth-Century Patent Medicines."
51. Holmes, "Currents and Counter-Currents in Medical Science," 25–27.

6. Cholera and the Emergence of the Gothic in American Medical Culture

1. For an introduction to the American cholera epidemics of the nineteenth century, see Rosenberg, *The Cholera Years.*
2. Grob, *The Deadly Truth,* 104–8.
3. "Progress of the Indian Cholera," *Daily National Intelligencer,* May 28, 1831.
4. "Foreign News," *Observer and Telegraph,* Jan. 27, 1831.
5. The response of European nations to the cholera epidemic is most fully examined in Baldwin, *Contagion and the State.*
6. "Cholera Morbus," *Globe,* July 6, 1831.
7. Baldwin, *Contagion and the State,* 43–52.
8. Ibid., 60–69. Sean Burrell and Geoffrey Gill argue that the Liverpool cholera riots of 1832 were prompted by a different set of factors, most significantly the belief among poorer residents that hospital staff were actually killing cholera sufferers and selling their bodies for dissection. Burrell and Gill, "The Liverpool Cholera Epidemic."
9. Baldwin, *Contagion and the State,* 69–71, 78–84.
10. Ibid., 92, 101.
11. Ibid., 93–110. See also Kelly, "'Not from the College.'"
12. "Cholera Morbus," *Daily National Journal,* Aug. 18, 1831.

13. "First Appearance and Progress of the Cholera at Moscow," *Globe*, Aug. 31, 1831.
14. "Intemperance and the Cholera," *Vermont Chronicle*, Sept. 23, 1831.
15. "Latest from England," *Boston Courier*, April 19, 1832.
16. "The Cholera," *United States' Telegraph*, Nov. 29, 1831.
17. "The Epidemic Cholera," *Daily National Intelligencer*, June 19, 1832.
18. *Report of the Commission Appointed by the Sanitary Board*, 1–8.
19. Ibid., 9–10.
20. Ibid. 10–11, 14.
21. *Reports of Hospital Physicians*, 14.
22. Ibid., 15, 93.
23. Ibid., 41, 44.
24. "The Cholera," *Daily National Intelligencer*, July 6, 1832; "The Cholera," *Boston Courier*, July 9, 1832.
25. "Doctors, MAURAN, WEBB & TOBEY, Who Were Recently Sent by the City Authority, to Visit the City of New-York," *Providence Patriot, Columbian Phenix*, July 14, 1832.
26. *Report of the Commission Appointed by the Sanitary Board*, 14, 18.
27. Ibid., 14.
28. Ibid., 19.
29. Ibid., 19–20.
30. Webster, *A Brief History of Epidemic and Pestilential Diseases*, 2:78–134.
31. Quoted in Apel, *Feverish Bodies, Enlightened Minds*, 55. On Webster's contributions to this yellow fever investigation more generally, see Apel, *Feverish Bodies, Enlightened Minds*, 35–64. See also Caldwell, "A Semi-Annual Oration on the Origins of Pestilential Diseases."
32. "Cholera in New-York," *New-York Spectator*, July 6, 1832.
33. "Desultory Remarks upon Cholera," *New-York Spectator*, July 13, 1832.
34. See Mukharji, "The 'Cholera Cloud' in the Nineteenth-Century 'British World.'"
35. Halttunen, *Murder Most Foul*.
36. Ibid., 62.
37. "The Cholera Morbus," *Providence Patriot, Columbian Phenix*, Aug. 10, 1831.
38. "The Cholera Morbus," *United States' Telegraph*, Aug. 15, 1831; "Communication," *United States' Telegraph*, Aug. 18, 1831.
39. "The Cholera," *Carolina Observer*, June 26, 1832.
40. "Popular Astronomy," *Macon Telegraph*, Aug. 20, 1831.
41. "The Cholera," *New England Weekly Review*, Sept. 12, 1831.
42. "The Cholera," *Liberator*, March 3, 1832; "Cholera," *Scioto Gazette*, June 27, 1832.
43. "Approach of Cholera," *Macon Telegraph*, June 27, 1832.
44. *Report of the Commission Appointed by the Sanitary Board*, 9.
45. "Effects of Fear," *Cherokee Phoenix, and Indians' Advocate*, Jan. 14, 1832.

46. Samuel Stevens, "The Cholera Morbus," *United States' Telegraph*, Jan. 16, 1832.
47. "A Cholera Subject Buried Alive," *Maryland Gazette*, March 29, 1832.
48. *Vermont Chronicle*, Aug. 26, 1831.
49. "Miscellaneous," *Liberator*, June 23, 1832.
50. "Description of the Cholera in Russia," *Arkansas Gazette*, Oct. 5, 1831.
51. "Symptoms of the Cholera as They Have Appeared in England," *Macon Telegraph*, Feb. 18, 1832.
52. "We Deem the Following Well Worthy the Attention of the Public," *Providence Patriot, Columbian Phenix*, June 23, 1832.
53. "Miscellaneous," *Liberator*, June 23, 1832.
54. "A Walk through a Cholera Hospital," *New-York Spectator*, June 19, 1832.
55. Brown, "Walstein's School of History," 333, 334.
56. Carey, *A Short Account of the Malignant Fever*.
57. See Hedges, "Benjamin Rush"; Levine, "The American Novel Begins"; and Hagenbüchle, "American Literature and the Nineteenth-Century Crisis in Epistemology."
58. Altschuler, *The Medical Imagination*, 78.
59. Gardiner, Review of *The Spy*, 281. See also Channing, Review of *Charles Brockden Brown*, and Foletta, *Coming to Terms with Democracy*, 110–11.
60. Leavitt, "Under the Shadow of Maternity."
61. For an introduction to puerperal fever, see Nuland, *The Doctors' Plague*. See also Peckham, "A Brief History of Puerperal Infection."
62. See Parsons, "Puerperal Fever." See also Nuland, *The Doctors' Plague*.
63. Quoted in Peckham, "A Brief History of Puerperal Infection," 199.
64. Holmes, "The Contagiousness of Puerperal Fever." See also Viets, "Oliver Wendell Holmes, Physician."
65. Meigs, *Obstetrics*, 635, 638, 639.
66. Ibid., 629, 633, 635.

7. Other Voices

1. Smith, "A Treatise on Fever," 364, and "On Malaria," 306, 321. See also Valenčius, *The Health of the Country*.
2. Henry, "Experiments on the Disinfecting Powers of Increased Temperatures." See also Henry, "Further Experiments on the Disinfecting Powers of Increased Temperatures."
3. "Plan of the Work," vi.
4. See Fulton and Thomson, "Benjamin Silliman," and Rossiter, "Benjamin Silliman and the Lowell Institute."
5. Mitchill, *Remarks on the Gaseous Oxyd of Azote*.

6. Brown, "An Account of the Pestilential Disease Which Prevailed at Boston." See also "Additional Account of the Pestilential Fever Which Prevailed at New London," and Channing, "An Account of the Pestilential Disease at New London."
7. Apel, *Feverish Bodies, Enlightened Minds*, 67.
8. "Respiration of Oxygen Gas"; Hare, "A New Process for Nitrous Ether," 326; Oliver, "On the Hydrocyanie"; Miller, "On the Use of Phosphoric Acid."
9. Carpenter, "Carpenter's Saratoga Powders." Other examples include "Some Experiments and Remarks on Several Species and Variations of Cinchona Bark," "Observations and Experiments on Opium," "Observations on a New Variety of Peruvian Bark," and "Notice of the Vesicating Principle of Cantharides."
10. Wood, "Notice of the Dispensatory of the United States of America."
11. Ibid., 152; "Announcement of the Founding of the Philadelphia College of Pharmacy."
12. "Address Delivered by the President, Daniel B. Smith," 255, 242. See also Higby, "Professionalism and the Nineteenth-Century American Pharmacist."
13. "Review of the *Journal of the Philadelphia College of Pharmacy*," 174.
14. Sonnedecker, "The Founding Period of the U.S. Pharmacopeia: II"; Sonnedecker, "The Founding Period of the U. S. Pharmacopeia: III."
15. "Review of *The Pharmacopeia of the United States of America*, Second Edition," 317, 336.
16. Sonnedecker, "The Founding Period of the U. S. Pharmacopeia: III."
17. "Review of *The Pharmacopeia of the United States of America, Washington 1830*," 71.
18. "Address Delivered by the President, Daniel B. Smith," 251; "Address Delivered to the Graduates by Henry Troth," 267.
19. "Article VI—Patent Medicines." See also Griffenhagen and Young, "Old English Patent Medicines," and Griffenhagen, "Early American Drug Containers."
20. "Article VI—Patent Medicines," 30; Griffenhagen and Young, "Old English Patent Medicines."
21. Estes, "The Pharmacology of Nineteenth-Century Patent Medicines"; Rothstein, *American Physicians in the Nineteenth Century*, 158–59; Burnham, *Health Care in America*, 81–83.
22. Griffenhagen and Young, "Old English Patent Medicines," 219, 220.
23. See Thomson, *A Narrative*. See also Rothstein, *American Physicians in the Nineteenth Century*, 125–51, and Haller, *Medical Protestants*, 31–65. On the role of herbal medicines and "root doctors" within southern slave communities, see Fett, *Working Cures*, 60–83.
24. Thomson, *A Narrative*, 25–26.
25. Ibid., 42.
26. Fillmore, "Samuel Thomson and His Effect."
27. Ibid. See also Berman, "The Thomsonian Movement."
28. See Rothstein, *American Physicians in the Nineteenth Century*, 125–51; Haller, *Medical Protestants*, 31–65; Berman, "The Thomsonian Movement"; and Klaw, "Belly My Grizzle." After obtaining a patent for his remedies, first available in 1813, licensed agents

offered individuals the right to practice Thomson's system within their family for just twenty dollars; for one hundred dollars people could buy the right to practice Thomsonian medicine on nonfamily members and even charge a fee.

29. For an introduction to the Second Great Awakening, see Hatch, *The Democratization of American Christianity*. On the codification movement, see Foletta, *Coming to Terms with Democracy*, 167–72.
30. Thomson, *A Narrative*, 39.
31. Estes, "The Shakers and Their Proprietary Medicines."
32. Thomson, *A Narrative*.
33. Ibid., 50, 66.
34. Ibid., 74, 91.
35. Ibid., 162.
36. Berman, "The Thomsonian Movement."
37. During the first third of the century many states conferred licensing authority on state medical societies. In a few, nonlicensed practitioners were only fined, but in many they were not allowed to pursue uncollected fees in court. See Rothstein, *American Physicians in the Nineteenth Century*, 144–51, 332–39; Haller, *Medical Protestants*, 31–65; and Dykstra, "The Medical Profession."
38. Hamilton, "Mercury and Water."
39. Buerki, "The Historical Development of an Ethic," 56, 57; Dykstra, "The Medical Profession," 405.
40. Rothstein, *American Physicians in the Nineteenth Century*, 144–51; Haller, *Medical Protestants*, 31–65.
41. The best introduction to homeopathy is Samuel Hahnemann's original text *Organon of Medicine*. See also Haller, *The History of American Homeopathy*, and Rothstein, *American Physicians in the Nineteenth Century*, 152–74.
42. Hahnemann, *Organon of Medicine*, 43, 65–70.
43. Ibid., 148–61.
44. Ibid., 234–42; Holmes, *Homeopathy and Its Kindred Delusions*.
45. Hahnemann, *Organon of Medicine*, preface, 21.
46. Ibid., 6, 13.
47. Ibid., 18; Cathrall, *Memoir on the Analysis of the Black Vomit*.
48. See Rogers, "The Proper Place of Homeopathy," 183.
49. See Haller, *Medical Protestants*, 139–98.
50. Parascandola, "The Emergence of Pharmaceutical Science."
51. Stover and Der Marderosian, "The Philadelphia College of Pharmacy."
52. Buerki, "Reception of the Germ Theory of Disease."
53. Cowen, "Pharmacists and Physicians."

8. Voices Ignored

1. On Nott's life and thought, see Horsman, *Josiah Nott of Mobile*.
2. Nott, "Yellow Fever Contrasted with Bilious Fever."
3. Nott, "The Epidemic Yellow Fever of Mobile."
4. See McMahon, "Beyond Therapeutics."
5. Finger, *The Contagious City*, 127–30.
6. On Philadelphia's more rigorous quarantine measures at Tinicum Island, see Barnes, *Lazaretto*.
7. For the standard explanation for the geographical migration of the disease, see Pierce and Writer, *Yellow Jack*, 47–59. James Goodyear offers a very different explanation in "The Sugar Connection."
8. The following discussion of New Orleans's distinctive adaptation to yellow fever draws heavily on Olivarius, *Necropolis*.
9. Ibid., 86.
10. Ibid., 14.
11. See Humphreys, *Yellow Fever and the South*, and Olivarius, *Necropolis*.
12. Williams, "An Account of the Yellow Fever Which Prevailed at Rodney, Mississippi," 36.
13. Lewis, "Sketch of the Yellow Fever of Mobile," 282.
14. Ibid., 285.
15. Hort, "Report of the Board of Health on the Sanitary Condition," 469.
16. Fenner, "An Account of the Yellow Fever That Prevailed in New Orleans."
17. Lewis, "An Extraordinary Case of Yellow Fever."
18. Cooke, "Practical Remarks on the Epidemic of Yellow Fever."
19. Beugnot, "An Essay on Yellow Fever," 12, 14, 19; *Federal Gazette*, Sept. 13, 1793.
20. Humphreys, *Yellow Fever and the South*, 17–76.
21. De Valetti and Logan, "A Report on the Yellow Fever"; Stone, "Report on the Origins of Yellow Fever."
22. De Valetti and Logan, "A Report on the Yellow Fever," 243.
23. Massie, "Observations on Yellow Fever," 37. Katherine Arner more fully describes the way in which anti-contagionists associated contagionism with "old world" fallacies. Concomitantly, local miasmatic theories took on nationalist connotations, a form of resistance to cultural imperialism. See Arner, "Making Yellow Fever American."
24. Stone, "Report on the Origins of Yellow Fever."
25. Cooke, "Practical Remarks on the Epidemic of Yellow Fever."
26. Humphreys, "Appendix II: Yellow Fever since 1793," 185.
27. Nott, "Yellow Fever Contrasted with Bilious Fever," 564–65, 571–72.
28. Ibid., 589. Texts and articles that exaggerate Nott's contributions include Harwood and James, *Entomology in Human and Animal Health*; Horsfall, *Medical Entomology*; and Service, "A Short History of Early Medical Entomology." See also Chernin, "Josiah Clark Nott, Insects and Yellow Fever."

29. Wilson, *The Invisible World*, 141–75, 148, 155 (quotations).
30. The following discussion of the microscope and its pioneers relies heavily on Wilson, *The Invisible World*, and Ruestow, *The Microscope in the Dutch Republic*.
31. Ball, "The Early History of the Compound Microscope."
32. Ibid.; Cassedy, "The Microscope in American Medical Science"; Hooke quoted in Wilson, *The Invisible World*, 221.
33. Woodruff, "The Advent of the Microscope at Yale College"; Cassedy, "The Microscope in American Medical Science."
34. Wilson, *The Invisible World*, 112.
35. Ibid., 234.
36. Ibid., 41.
37. Bradley, *The Plague at Marseilles Consider'd*, 46.
38. Holland, *Medical Notes and Reflections*, 342, 344, 349.
39. Crawford, "Remarks on Quarantine Suggested by Dr. Caldwell's Oration," 1:404; 2:40.
40. Ibid., 1:314, 301, 325. See also Peller, "Walter Reed, C. Finlay, and Their Predecessors."
41. Riddell, *Memoir on the Nature of Miasm and Contagion*, 4–6, 12, 19.
42. Nott, "Yellow Fever Contrasted with Bilious Fever," 567.
43. Ibid., 593–94.
44. Harris, *A Treatise on Some of the Insects of New England*, 2.
45. See Stroud, *Thomas Say*.
46. Quoted in ibid., 209.
47. Say, *American Entomology*, iv; Stroud, *Thomas Say*, 46.
48. Say, *American Entomology*, 36, 77, 109–10.
49. Horsman, *Josiah Nott of Mobile*, 5–20.
50. Benjamin Rush to Julia Rush, Sept. 25, 1793, in Rush, *Letters of Benjamin Rush*, 2:683–84.
51. Herschthal, "Antislavery Science in the Early Republic."
52. Hogarth, *Medicalizing Blackness*.
53. Fett, *Working Cures*, 15–36.
54. Savitt, "The Use of Blacks for Medical Experimentation." See also Savitt, *Medicine and Slavery*, 281–307, and Willoughby, *Masters of Health*.
55. Fitzhugh, *Sociology for the South*.
56. Nott, *Two Lectures on the Natural History of the Caucasian and Negro Races*. See also Horsman, *Race and Manifest Destiny*.
57. Nott, *Two Lectures on the Natural History of the Caucasian and Negro Races*, 29, 19, 34, 16. See also Nott, "The Mulatto."
58. Nott, *Two Lectures on the Natural History of the Caucasian and Negro Races*, 36.

9. After a Century the Mystery Is Solved

1. On these developments, see Burnham, *Health Care in America*, especially 59–98; Warner, *Against the Spirit of the System*, 17–31; Ludmerer, *Learning to Heal;* Numbers, ed., *The Education of American Physicians;* and Rothstein, *American Physicians in the Nineteenth Century*. See also Atwater, "The Protracted Labor and Brief Life of a Country Medical School."
2. Rothstein, *American Physicians in the Nineteenth Century*, 97.
3. Ludmerer, *Learning to Heal*, 12; Rothstein, *American Physicians in the Nineteenth Century*, 113, 12.
4. Sappol, *A Traffic of Dead Bodies*, offers the most comprehensive treatment of the rising importance of anatomy instruction in American medical education and the resulting traffic in dead bodies.
5. Willoughby, *Masters of Health*, 78–80.
6. Sappol, *A Traffic of Dead Bodies*, 29–43.
7. Sappol, *A Traffic of Dead Bodies*, 4–5, 123–32; Blake, "Anatomy," 36–38; Blake, "The Development of American Anatomy Acts."
8. Sappol, *A Traffic of Dead Bodies*, 113, 115; Breeden, "Body Snatchers and Anatomy Professors."
9. Sappol, *A Traffic of Dead Bodies*, 74–98. Ponce challenges this analysis in "'They Increase in Beauty and Elegance,'" 333–34.
10. Ponce, "'They Increase in Beauty and Elegance,'" 345–57.
11. See Longo, "Obstetrics and Gynecology."
12. "Report of the Committee Appointed under the Fourth Resolution of the National Medical Convention."
13. Ibid., 71.
14. Ibid., 63.
15. Warner, *Against the Spirit of the System*. See also Weiner and Sauter, "The City of Paris and the Rise of Clinical Medicine." Warner also points out that assessments of the Paris School have been divided between those emphasizing its constructive contributions to medical science and those more critical of the resulting shift in "clinical attention from individual sick people as the focus of healing to disease entities as the objects of research" (4). The former position is maintained by Erwin H. Ackerknecht in *Medicine at the Paris Hospital;* the latter was argued by Michel Foucault in *The Birth of the Clinic*. Seeming to support Foucault's analysis, many American students returned to the United States impressed by French methods of diagnosis and education but critical of the care French doctors gave their patients—their "valuation of knowledge above healing." Warner, *Against the Spirit of the System*, 10.
16. Warner, *Against the Spirit of the System*, especially 32–75.
17. Ibid.
18. Freemon, *Gangrene and Glory*, 25, 142.
19. For a more complete review of ether's development, see Rutkow, *Seeking the Cure*, 51–60.

20. Albin, "The Use of Anesthetics during the Civil War."
21. Gilchrist, "Disease and Infection in the American Civil War"; Freemon, *Gangrene and Glory*, 48–49; Ludmerer, *Learning to Heal*, 9–10; Bollet, "Amputations in the Civil War," 64–65.
22. Hasegawa, "Southern Resources, Southern Medicines"; Freemon, *Gangrene and Glory*, 48.
23. See Humphreys, *Marrow of Tragedy*, 20–26.
24. Flannery, "Civil War Pharmacy and Medicine"; Freemon, *Gangrene and Glory*.
25. Hamilton, "Mercury and Water."
26. Shryock, "A Medical Perspective on the Civil War"; Gilchrist, "Disease and Infection in the American Civil War," 258.
27. See Devine, *Learning from the Wounded*.
28. Ibid., 22.
29. Ibid., 83–86, 94–131.
30. Ibid.
31. See Humphreys, *Yellow Fever and the South;* Pierce and Writer, *Yellow Jack;* and *Report of a Committee of the Associate Members of the Sanitary Commission*.
32. Pierce and Writer, *Yellow Jack*, 69, 71.
33. See Rutkow, *Seeking the Cure*, 64–71.
34. Ibid., 67.
35. For an introduction to Koch's life and work, see Adler, *Robert Koch*. See also Gehlbach, *American Plagues*, 111–12. Perhaps the best indicator of America's comparative theoretical and practical stasis is that its greatest contribution during these years was the publication of the *Index Medicus*, a monthly catalog of all new medical publications, the vast majority from Europe. See Burnham, *Health Care in America*, 99–102.
36. Adler, *Robert Koch*, 40–45; Codell, "The Koch-Pasteur Dispute."
37. Adler, *Robert Koch*, 45–48.
38. Ibid.
39. King, "Dr. Koch's Postulates"; Adler, *Robert Koch*, 50–51.
40. For an introduction to Finlay and his role in solving this etiological mystery, see Del Regato, "Carlos Juan Finlay." See also Pierce and Writer, *Yellow Jack*, 75–82. Nancy Stepan explains the twenty-year gap between Finlay's suggestive research and its wider embrace in "The Interplay between Socio-Economic Factors and Medical Science."
41. McNeill, *Mosquito Empires*, 259, 300.
42. Quoted in Espinosa, *Epidemic Invasions*, 28. See also Espinosa "The Threat from Havana."
43. Grob, *The Deadly Truth*, 194–95; Espinosa, *Epidemic Invasions*, 33–46.
44. Pierce and Writer, *Yellow Jack*, 103, 109.
45. Ibid., 83–86.
46. On Reed's life, see Bean, *Walter Reed*. For a brief introduction to his early life, see Fink, "Before Yellow Fever and Cuba."

47. Peller, "Walter Reed, C. Finlay, and Their Predecessors."
48. The appropriateness of these experiments on human subjects has been debated ever since. See, for example, Bean, "Walter Reed and the Ordeal of Human Experiments."
49. Schultz, "Photo Quiz—Henry Rose Carter."
50. Espinosa, *Epidemic Invasions*, 63–70.
51. Adler, *Robert Koch*, 214–20; Maulitz, "Pathology," 135–37.
52. In addition to Devine, *Learning from the Wounded,* see Gossel, "Pasteur, Koch and American Bacteriology." On the more general transformation of American medicine and medical practice, see Burnham, *Health Care in America,* especially 141–87.

BIBLIOGRAPHY

Primary Sources

"An Account of the Effects of Copious Blood-Letting, in a Case of Difficult Parturition. By Dr. John Spence in a Letter to Dr. Benjamin Rush." *Philadelphia Medical Museum* 3, no. 3 (1807): 174–75.

"An Account of the Efficacy of Salivation in Curing Pulmonary Consumption, in a Letter from Dr. Maxwell McDowell of Yorktown, in Pennsylvania, to Benjamin Rush." *Philadelphia Medical Museum* 2, no. 4 (1806): 400.

"An Account of the Good Effects of Copious Blood Letting in the Cure of a Hemorrhage of the Lungs, in a Letter from the Rev. Dr. Samuel Smith to Benjamin Rush, March 19, 1798." *Philadelphia Medical Museum* 2, no. 1 (1806): 1–5.

"An Account of the Introduction of the Vaccine Disease into the Isles of France and Reunion. In a Letter to the Editor from M. Laborde, M.D." *Philadelphia Medical and Physical Journal* 2, no.1 (1806): 71–75.

"An Account of Two Cases of Dropsy Cured by the Loss of Blood, Extracted from a Letter from Dr. James Wallace, from Fauquier County, in Virginia, to Dr. Benjamin Rush." *Philadelphia Medical Museum* 2, no. 4 (1806): 401–2.

"Additional Account of the Pestilential Fever Which Prevailed at New London; Letter from Dr. Coit to Dr. Mitchill." *Medical Repository* 2 (1798–99): 407–8.

"Address Delivered by the President, Daniel B. Smith, September 24, 1829." *Journal of the Philadelphia College of Pharmacy* 1, no. 4 (1830): 241–62.

"Address Delivered to the Graduates by Henry Troth, Esq." *Journal of the Philadelphia College of Pharmacy* 2, no. 4 (1831): 257–71.

Alibert, J. L. "A Treatise on Malignant Intermittents." *Medical Repository* 5 (1807): 51–54.

Allen, Richard, and Absalom Jones. *A Narrative of the Proceedings of the Black People during the Late Awful Calamity in Philadelphia*. Philadelphia: William Woodward, 1794.

"Announcement of the Founding of the Philadelphia College of Pharmacy." *Pharmacy in History* 50, no. 1 (2008): 27–29.

"Article VI—Patent Medicines." *Journal of the Philadelphia College of Pharmacy* 5, no. 4 (1834): 20–31.

Beguerie, J. M. "Histoire de la fievre qui a regnè sur la flotilla Françoise en 1802." *Medical Repository* 4 (1807): 290–94.

Beugnot, J. F. "An Essay on Yellow Fever, Read before the Louisiana Medico-Chirurgical Society, Sept. 1843." *New Orleans Medical and Surgical Journal* 1, no 1 (1844–45): 1–28.

Bradley, Richard. *The Plague at Marseilles Consider'd.* London: W. Mears, 1721.

Brown, Charles Brockden. *Arthur Mervyn; or, Memoir of the Year 1793, with Related Texts.* Edited by Philip Barnard and Stephen Shapiro. Indianapolis: Hackett, 2008.

———. "Walstein's School of History. From the German Krants of Gotha." *Monthly Magazine and American Review* 1, no. 5 (1799): 335–38. Reprinted in Charles Brockden Brown, *Arthur Mervyn; or, Memoir of the Year 1793, with Related Texts,* ed. Philip Barnard and Stephen Shapiro (Indianapolis: Hackett, 2008), 331–45.

Brown, John. *The Elements of Medicine of John Brown, M.D.* London: J. Johnson, 1795. The work was published in Latin in 1780 and first translated into English in 1788.

Brown, Samuel. "An Account of the Pestilential Disease Which Prevailed at Boston, 1798." *Medical Repository* 2, no. 4 (1798–99): 390–97.

Browne, Joseph. "Treatise on the Yellow Fever." *Medical Repository* 1, no. 4 (1797–98): 547–50.

Caldwell, Charles. "A Semi-Annual Oration on the Origins of Pestilential Diseases, Delivered before the Academy of Medicine of Philadelphia, December 17, 1798." *Medical Repository* 3, no. 1 (1799–1800): 58–61.

Carey, Mathew. *A Short Account of the Malignant Fever Lately Prevalent in Philadelphia.* Philadelphia: Mathew Carey, 1793.

Carpenter, George W. "Carpenter's Saratoga Powders." *American Journal of Science and Arts* 16, no. 2 (1829): 369–70.

———. "Notice of the Vesicating Principle of Cantharides." *American Journal of Science and Arts* 21, no. 1 (1832): 69–70.

———. "Observations and Experiments on Opium." *American Journal of Science and Arts* 13, no. 1 (1828): 7–32.

———. "Observations on a New Variety of Peruvian Bark." *American Journal of Science and Arts* 20, no. 1 (1831): 52–56.

———. "Some Experiments and Remarks on Several Species and Variations of Cinchona Bark." *American Journal of Science and Arts* 9, no. 2 (1825): 363–65.

"Case of Superfoetation Communicated by Dr. Farquhar." *Philadelphia Medical Museum* 2, no. 3 (1806): 316.

Cathrall, Isaac. *A Medical Sketch of the Synochus Maligna; or, Malignant Contagious Fever; as It Lately Appeared in the City of Philadelphia: To Which Is Added, Some Account of the Morbid Appearances That Appear after Death, on Dissection.* Philadelphia: T. Dobson, 1794.

———. *Memoir on the Analysis of the Black Vomit, Ejected in the Last Stage of the Yellow Fever.* Philadelphia: R. Folwell, 1800.

Channing, Edward Tyrrel. "Review of Charles Brockden Brown." *North American Review* 9 (1819): 58–77.

Channing, Henry. "An Account of the Pestilential Disease at New London, 1798." *Medical Repository* 2, no. 4 (1798–99): 402–4.

The Charter, Constitution, and By Laws of the College of Physicians of Philadelphia. Philadelphia: Zachariah Poulson, 1790.

Chisholm, Colin. *An Essay on the Malignant Pestilential Fever Introduced into the West Indies from Boullam on the Coast of Guinea.* London: C. Dilly, 1795.

Church, John. "Observations on Mr. Goldson's Pamphlet." *Philadelphia Medical Museum* 1, no. 3 (1805): 323–26.

Clark, G. "Case of Extra-Uterine Gestation." *Philadelphia Medical Museum* 2, no. 2 (1806): 292–95.

"College of Physicians to Governor Mifflin." *Medical Repository* 1, no. 3 (1797–98): 343–48.

Cooke, T. A. "Practical Remarks on the Epidemic of Yellow Fever, Which Prevailed at Opelousas in the Years 1837, '39, and '42." *New Orleans Medical and Surgical Journal* 3, no. 1 (1846–47): 27–40.

Crawford, John. "Remarks on Quarantine Suggested by Dr. Caldwell's Oration." In *The Observatory and Repertory of Original and Selected Essays in Verse and Prose on Topics of Polite Literature,* 2 vols., edited by Eliza Anderson, 1:248–55, 262–66, 283–86, 299–302, 314–18, 325–30, 344–48, 373–77, 404–8; 2:7–10, 20–25, 33–39, 49–54, 65–70. Baltimore: J. Robinson, 1807.

Currie William. *A Description of the Malignant, Infectious Fever, Prevailing at Present in Philadelphia: With an Account of the Means to Prevent Infection and the Remedies and Method of Treatment, Which Have Been Found Most Successful.* Philadelphia: T. Dobson, 1793.

———. *A Dissertation on the Autumnal Remitting Fever.* Philadelphia: Peter Stewart, 1789.

———. *An Historical Account of the Climate and Diseases of the United States.* Philadelphia: T. Dobson, 1792.

———. "Notice of the Yellow Fever." *Philadelphia Medical and Physical Journal* 2, no. 1 (1805): 45–49.

———. *Of the Cholera.* Philadelphia: William T. Palmer, 1798.

Currie, William, and Isaac Cathrall. *Facts and Observations, Relative to the Origin, Progress and Nature of the Fever, Which Prevailed in Certain Parts of the City and Districts of Philadelphia, in the Summer and Autumn of the Present Year (1802). To Which Is Added, a Summary of the Rise and Progress of the Disease in Wilmington.* Philadelphia: William W. Woodward, 1802.

Danielson, L., and E. Mann. "The History of a Singular and Very Mortal Disease, Which Lately Made Its Appearance in Medfield." *Medical and Agricultural Register* 1, no. 5 (1806): 65–69.

De Valetti, C., and Thomas M. Logan. "A Report on the Yellow Fever That Recently Prevailed at Woodville, Mississippi." *New Orleans Medical and Surgical Journal* 1, no. 3 (1844–45): 237–43.

Deveze, Jean. *An Enquiry into and Observations upon the Causes and Effects of the Epidemic, Which Raged in Philadelphia from the Month of August towards the Middle of December, 1793.* Philadelphia: Parent, 1794.

Dewees, William. "An Attempt to Explain Why More Children Live That Are Born at the Seventh, Than at the Eighth Month of Pregnancy." *Philadelphia Medical Museum* 2, no. 3 (1806): 274–80.

———. "Case of a Ruptured Uterus." *Philadelphia Medical Museum* 2, no. 4 (1806): 411–17.

———. "On the Efficacy of Blood-Letting in Rigidity of the Os Externum." *Philadelphia Medical Museum* 2, no. 1 (1806): 27–30.

"Dr. Drysdale's History of the Yellow Fever at Baltimore—Letter VI." *Philadelphia Medical Museum* 1, no. 2 (1805): 140–49.

"Dr. John Spence to the Editor." *Philadelphia Medical Museum* 1, no. 4 (1805): 401–6.
"Dr. Morton's Summary of the History of the Continued Fever in England from 1658 to 1691." *Medical Repository* 1 (1797–98): 56–63.
Drinker, Elizabeth. *The Diary of Elizabeth Drinker*. Edited by Elaine Forman Crane. 3 vols. Boston: Northeastern University Press, 1991.
Elmer, J. "Case of Mortification and Separation of the Body of the Uterus; Also an Account of a Monstrous Birth." *Philadelphia Medical Museum* 2, no. 1 (1806): 70–72.
"Extract from the Asiatic Annual Register." *Philadelphia Medical Museum* 2, no. 2 (1806): 434–40.
"Facts and Observations, Chiefly Relative to the Yellow Fever, as It Appeared, at Different Times, in Charleston, South Carolina, in a Letter from Dr. Tudor Smith to Dr. William Currie." *Philadelphia Medical and Physical Journal* 2, no. 1 (1805): 21–34.
Fenner, E. D. "An Account of the Yellow Fever That Prevailed in New Orleans in the Year 1846." *New Orleans Medical and Surgical Journal* 3, no. 4 (1846–47): 445–66.
"Fetus Found in the Abdomen of a Boy Fourteen Years of Age." *Philadelphia Medical Museum* 2, no. 2 (1806): 226–28.
Ffirth, Stubbins. *A Treatise on Malignant Fever with an Attempt to Prove Its Non-Contagious Nature*. Philadelphia: B. Graves, 1804.
Fitzhugh, George. *Sociology for the South; or, The Failure of Free Society*. Richmond, Va.: A. Morris, 1854.
Gardiner, William H. Review of *The Spy*. *North American Review* 15 (July 1822): 250–82.
Goldson, William. *Cases of Small Pox, Subsequent to Vaccination, with Facts and Observations, Read before the Medical Society, at Portsmouth, March 29th, 1804*. London: W. Woodward, 1804.
Hahnemann, Samuel. *Organon of Medicine*. 1833; New Delhi, India: B. Jain, 2018.
Hardie, James. *An Account of the Rise, Progress, and Termination of the Malignant Fever Lately Prevalent in Philadelphia. Briefly Stated from Authentic Documents*. Philadelphia: Benjamin Johnson, 1793.
Hare, Robert. "A New Process for Nitrous Ether." *American Journal of Science* 2, no. 2 (1820): 326–27.
Harris, Dr. "History of a Fatal Case of Hydrocephalus." *Philadelphia Medical Museum* 2, no. 4 (1806): 384–99.
Harris, Thaddeus William. *A Treatise on Some of the Insects of New England Which Are Injurious to Vegetation*. Cambridge, Mass: John Owen, 1842.
Hazen Edward. "The Druggist and the Apothecary" (1841). *Pharmacy in History* 39, no. 2 (1997): 73–75.
Henry, William. "Experiments on the Disinfecting Powers of Increased Temperatures, with a View to the Suggestion of a Substitute for Quarantine." *American Journal of Science and Arts* 21, no. 2 (1832): 392–99.
———. "Further Experiments on the Disinfecting Powers of Increased Temperatures." *American Journal of Science and Arts* 22, no.1 (1832): 111–21.
Holland, Henry. *Medical Notes and Reflections*. Philadelphia: Haswell, Barrington, and Haswell, 1839.
Holmes, Oliver Wendell. "The Contagiousness of Puerperal Fever." *New England Quarterly Journal of Medicine* 1 (1843): 503–30.

———. "Currents and Counter-Currents in Medical Science, an Address Delivered before the Massachusetts Medical Society, at the Annual Meeting, May 30, 1860." In *Currents and Counter-Currents in Medical Science, with Other Addresses and Essays*, 1–50. Boston: Ticknor and Fields, 1861.

———. *Homeopathy and Its Kindred Delusions: Two Lectures Delivered before the Boston Society for the Diffusion of Useful Knowledge*. Boston: William D. Ticknor, 1842.

Hort, W. P. "Report of the Board of Health on the Sanitary Condition of the City of New Orleans, during the Year 1846, and the Means of Improving It." *New Orleans Medical and Surgical Journal* 3, no. 4 (1846–47): 467–78.

Koch, Adrienne, ed. *The American Enlightenment: The Shaping of the American Experiment and a Free Society*. New York: George Braziller, 1965.

"Letter from Doctor James Mann on the Treatment of Croup or Rattles or Quincy." *Medical and Agricultural Register* 1, no. 13 (1807): 209–11.

"Letter from the College of Physicians to Governor Mifflin." *Medical Repository* 1, no. 3 (1797–98): 412–14.

Lewis, J. Hampden. "An Extraordinary Case of Yellow Fever, Accompanied with Gangrene of the Leg." *New Orleans Medical and Surgical Journal* 1, no. 5 (1844–45): 409–31.

Lewis, P. H. "Sketch of the Yellow Fever of Mobile with a Brief Analysis of the Epidemic of 1843." *New Orleans Medical and Surgical Journal* 1, no. 4 (1844–45): 281–305.

Massie, J. C. "Observations on Yellow Fever." *New Orleans Medical and Surgical Journal* 9, no. 1 (1852–53): 35–40.

Mease, James. "Account of the Efficacy of the External Application of the Geranium Maculatum, in Stopping Hemorrhage." *Philadelphia Medical Museum* 3, no. 3 (1807): 145–50.

"Medical and Philosophical Register." *Philadelphia Medical Museum* 1, no. 2 (1805): 224–25.

"Medical and Philosophical Register." *Philadelphia Medical Museum* 1, no. 3 (1805): 353–54.

"Medical Extracts." *Medical and Agricultural Register* 1, no. 5 (1806): 69–72.

"Medical Register." *Philadelphia Medical Museum* 1, no. 2 (1805): 215–24.

Meigs, Charles. *Obstetrics: The Science and the Art*. 3rd edition. 1849; Philadelphia: Blanchard and Lea, 1856.

Miller, Caleb. "On the Use of Phosphoric Acid in Jaundice." *American Journal of Science* 4, no. 1 (1822): 162–63.

Mitchill, Samuel. *Remarks on the Gaseous Oxyd of Azote or of Nitrogene*. New York: T. and J. Swords, 1795.

Morgan, John. *A Discourse upon the Institution of Medical Schools in America*. Philadelphia: William Bradford, 1765.

———. *Doctor Morgan's Remarks on Dr. Shippen's Feeble Attempts to Vindicate Himself*. Philadelphia: David C. Claypoole, 1781.

———. *To the Citizens and Freemen of the United States of America*. Philadelphia: M. K. Goddard, 1778.

———. *A Vindication of His Public Character in the Station of Director General of the Military Hospitals and Physician in Chief to the American Army*. Boston: Powers and Willis, 1777.

Nassy, David de Isaac Cohen. *Observations on the Cause, Nature, and Treatment of the Epidemic Disorder, Prevalent in Philadelphia*. Philadelphia: Parker, 1793.

Nott, Josiah. "The Epidemic Yellow Fever of Mobile in 1853." *New Orleans Medical and Surgical Journal* 10 (1854): 571–83.

———. "The Mulatto, a Hybrid—Probable Extermination of the Two Races if the Whites and Blacks Are Allowed to Intermarry." *New Orleans Medical and Surgical Journal* 6, no. 11 (1843): 252–56.

———. *Two Lectures on the Natural History of the Caucasian and Negro Races*. Mobile, Ala.: Dade and Thompson, 1844.

———. "Yellow Fever Contrasted with Bilious Fever." *New Orleans Medical and Surgical Journal* 4, no. 5 (1847–48): 563–601.

"Observations on Certain Cases of Secondary Disease, Subsequent to the Measles, in a Letter to Benjamin Rush, March 9, 1805." *Philadelphia Medical Museum* 2, no. 3 (1806): 241–73.

"Observations on the Preceding Paper, in a Letter from Dr. William Currie to Dr. Tucker Harris." *Philadelphia Medical and Physical Journal* 2, no. 1 (1805): 34–45.

"Observations on Vaccination." *Philadelphia Medical Museum* 1, no 4 (1805): 434–36.

"Observations upon the Yellow Fever, in a Letter from Dr. George Davidson to James Mease." *Medical Repository* 1 (1797–98): 165–72.

Oliver, B. Lynde. "On the Hydrocyanie or Prussic Acid." *American Journal of Science* 3, no. 1 (1821): 182–87.

"On Malaria." *American Journal of Science and Arts* 17, no. 2 (1830): 300–328.

Pascalis-Ouvière, Felix. *An Account of the Contagious Epidemic Yellow Fever, Which Prevailed in Philadelphia in the Summer and Autumn of 1797; Comprising the Questions of Its Causes and Domestic Origin, Characters, Medical Treatment, and Preventatives*. Philadelphia: Snowden and M'Corkle, 1798.

"Plan of the Work." *American Journal of Science* 1, no. 1 (1818–19): v–vi.

Ramsey, David. *An Eulogium upon Benjamin Rush, M.D., Professor of the Institutes and Practice of Medicine and of Clinical Practice in the University of Pennsylvania*. Philadelphia: Bradford and Inskeep, 1813.

Report of a Committee of the Associate Members of the Sanitary Commission, on the Subject of the Nature and Treatment of Yellow Fever. New York: W. C. Bryant, 1862.

Report of the Commission Appointed by the Sanitary Board of the City Councils, to Visit Canada, for the Investigation of the Epidemic Cholera, Prevailing in Montreal and Quebec. Philadelphia: Mifflin and Parry, 1832.

"Report of the Committee Appointed under the Fourth Resolution of the National Medical Convention, Which Assembled in New York, in May, 1846." in *Proceedings of the National Medical Convention held in New York, in May, 1846, and in Philadelphia, in May, 1847*, 63–77. Philadelphia: Collins, 1847.

Reports of Hospital Physicians, and Other Documents in Relation to the Epidemic Cholera of 1832. New York: New York Board of Health, 1832.

"Respiration of Oxygen Gas." *American Journal of Science* 1, no. 1 (1818–19): 95–96.

"Review of *An Inaugural Essay on Yellow Fever as It Appeared in This City (New York) in 1795* by Alexander Hosack, Jun." *Medical Repository* 1, no. 2 (1797–98): 224–31.

"Review of *Medical Inquiries and Observations: Containing an Account of the Bilious and Remitting Yellow Fever as It Appeared in the City of Philadelphia, in the Year 1794*." *Medical Repository* 1 (1797–98), no. 1: 79–85; no. 2: 206–11, no. 3: 337–43.

"Review of *Memoirs of the Yellow Fever* by William Currie." *Medical Repository* 2, no. 3 (1798–99): 312–14.

"Review of the *Journal of the Philadelphia College of Pharmacy.*" *American Journal of Science* 21, no. 1 (1832): 173–79.

"Review of *The Pharmacopeia of the United States of America*, Second Edition." *Journal of the Philadelphia College of Pharmacy* 2, no. 4 (1831): 315–36.

"Review of *The Pharmacopeia of the United States of America, Washington 1830.*" *Journal of the Philadelphia College of Pharmacy* 3, no. 1 (1832): 64–86.

Riddell, John L. *Memoir on the Nature of Miasm and Contagion.* Cincinnati: N. S. Johnson, 1836.

Rousseau, J. C. "More Proof of Vaccination's Effectiveness." *Philadelphia Medical Museum* 1, no. 4 (1805): 424–27.

Rush, Benjamin. *An Account of the Bilious Remitting Yellow Fever, as It Appeared in the City of Philadelphia in 1793.* Philadelphia: Thomas Dobson, 1793.

———. *An Address to the Inhabitants of the British Settlements in America upon Slave Keeping.* Philadelphia: John Dunlap, 1773.

———. *The Autobiography of Benjamin Rush.* Edited by George W. Corner. Princeton, N.J.: Princeton University Press, 1948.

———. *Benjamin Rush's Lectures on the Mind.* Edited by Eric T. Carlson, Jeffrey L. Wollock, and Patricia S. Noel. Philadelphia: American Philosophical Society, 1981.

———. "An Inquiry into the Natural History of Medicine among the Indians of North America." In Benjamin Rush, *Medical Inquiries and Observations,* 3rd edition, 4 vols., 1:101–69. Philadelphia: Hopkins and Earle, 1809.

———. "Lecture upon the Causes Which Have Retarded the Progress of Medicine." In *Sixteen Introductory Lectures, to Courses of Lectures upon the Institutes and Practice of Medicine,* 141–66. Philadelphia: Bradford and Innskeep, 1811.

———. "Letter of Dr. Rush and Others to Governor Mifflin." *Medical Repository* 1 (1797–98): 405–12.

———. *Letters of Benjamin Rush.* Edited by L. H. Butterfield. 2 vols. Princeton, N.J.: Princeton University Press, 1951.

———. *The New Method of Inoculating for the Smallpox—Delivered in a Lecture in the University of Pennsylvania, on the 20th of February, 1781.* Philadelphia: Charles Cist, 1781.

———. "Observations on the Duties of a Physician and the Methods of Improving Medicine, Delivered in the University of Pennsylvania, February 7, 1789." In Benjamin Rush, *Medical Inquiries and Observations,* 3rd edition, 4 vols., 1:433–56. Philadelphia: Hopkins and Earle, 1809.

———. "On the Duties of Patients to Their Physicians, November 7, 1808." In *Sixteen Introductory Lectures, to Courses of Lectures upon the Institutes and Practice of Medicine,* 318–39. Philadelphia: Bradford and Innskeep, 1811.

———. "On the Means of Acquiring Business and the Causes Which Prevent the Acquisition, and Occasion the Loss of It, in the Profession of Medicine, Delivered November 4, 1807." In *Sixteen Introductory Lectures, to Courses of Lectures upon the Institutes and Practice of Medicine,* 222–55. Philadelphia: Bradford and Innskeep, 1811.

Say, Thomas. *American Entomology; or, Descriptions of the Insects of North America.* Philadelphia: Mitchell and Ames, 1817.

Shattuck, George. "An Essay on the Influence of Air upon Animal Bodies." *Philadelphia Medical and Physical Journal* 3, no. 1 (1808): 3–17.

Smith, Elihu Hubbard. *The Diary of Elihu Hubbard Smith, 1771–1798.* Edited by James E. Cronin. Philadelphia: American Philosophical Society, 1973.

———. "The Plague of Athens." *Medical Repository of Critical Essays and Intelligence Relative to Physic, Surgery, Chemistry, and Natural History* 1, no. 1 (1797–98): 1–30.

Smith, Southwood. "A Treatise on Fever." *American Journal of Science and Arts* 19, no. 2 (1831): 363–65.

Smith, Thomas. "Facts and Observations Relative to the Bilious Remitting Fever of Loudon County in Virginia." *Philadelphia Medical and Physical Journal* 3, no. 1 (1806): 19–22.

Stearns, Samuel. *An Account of the Terrible Effects of the Pestilential Infection in the City of Philadelphia in 1793.* Providence: William Child, 1793.

Stone, C. H. "Report on the Origins of Yellow Fever in the Town of Woodville, Mississippi, in the summer of 1844." *New Orleans Medical and Surgical Journal* 1, no. 6 (1844–45): 520–36.

Thomson, Samuel. *A Narrative of the Life and Medical Discoveries of Samuel Thomson: Containing an Account of His System of Practice, and the Manner of Curing Disease with Vegetable Medicine.* Columbus, Ohio: J. Pike, 1835.

"Vaccine Inoculation: Statement of the Number of Persons Inoculated at the Society." *Philadelphia Medical Museum* 1, no. 4 (1805): 454–56.

Vaughan, John. "Account of Two Albinos." *Philadelphia Medical Museum* 2, no. 3 (1806): 284–86.

Watkins, T. "On the Utility of Spirit of Turpentine in a Severe Burn." *Philadelphia Medical Museum* 3, no. 1 (1807): 58–60.

Webster Noah. *A Brief History of Epidemic and Pestilential Diseases with the Principal Phenomena of the Physical World Which Precede Them and Accompany Them and Observations Deduced from the Facts Stated.* 2 vols. Hartford, Conn.: Hudson and Godwin, 1799.

———. *A Collection of Papers on the Subject of Bilious Fevers, Prevalent in the United States for a Few Years Past.* New York: Hopkins, Webb, 1796.

Wheaton, Dr. L. "A Brief Account of the Yellow Fever in Providence, Rhode Island." *Medical Repository* 4 (February–April 1807): 329–41.

Williams, William G. "An Account of the Yellow Fever Which Prevailed at Rodney, Mississippi, during the Autumn of 1843." *New Orleans Medical and Surgical Journal* 1, no. 1 (1844–45): 35–43.

Wood, George B. "Notice of the Dispensatory of the United States of America." *American Journal of Science and Arts* 24, no. 1 (1833): 151–60.

Newspapers

The Argus, or Greenleaf's New Daily Advertiser [New York]
Arkansas Gazette [Little Rock]
Boston Courier
Carolina Observer [Fayetteville, N.C.]
Cherokee Phoenix, and Indians' Advocate [New Echota, Ga.]
Commercial Advertiser [New York]
Daily National Intelligencer [Washington, D.C.]
Daily National Journal [Washington, D.C.]

Dunlap's American Daily Advertiser [Philadelphia]
Federal Gazette [Philadelphia]
Gazette of the United States [Philadelphia]
General Advertiser [Philadelphia]
Globe [Washington, D.C.]
Liberator [Boston]
Macon Telegraph [Macon, Ga.]
The Mail or Claypoole's Daily Advertiser [Philadelphia]
Maryland Gazette [Annapolis]
New England Weekly Review [Hartford, Conn.]
New-York Spectator
Observer and Telegraph [Hudson, Ohio]
Pennsylvania Chronicle [Philadelphia]
Pennsylvania Evening Post [Philadelphia]
Pennsylvania Federal Gazette [Philadelphia]
Pennsylvania Packet [Philadelphia]
Philadelphia Gazette and Universal Daily Advertiser
Porcupine's Gazette [Philadelphia]
Providence Patriot, Columbian Phenix [Providence, R.I.]
Scioto Gazette [Chillicothe, Ohio]
United States' Telegraph [Washington, D.C.]
Vermont Chronicle [Bellows Falls]

Secondary Works Cited

Abrams, Jeanne E. *Revolutionary Medicine: The Founding Fathers and Mothers in Sickness and Health.* New York: New York University Press, 2013.

Ackerknecht, Erwin H. "Anticontagionism between 1821 and 1867." *Bulletin of the History of Medicine* 22 (1948): 562–93.

———. *Medicine at the Paris Hospital, 1794–1848.* Baltimore: Johns Hopkins University Press, 1967.

Adler, Richard. *Robert Koch and American Bacteriology.* Jefferson, N.C.: McFarland, 2016.

Albin, Maurice S. "The Use of Anesthetics during the Civil War, 1861–1865." *Pharmacy in History* 42, nos. 3–4 (2000): 99–114.

Alchon, Suzanne Austin. *A Pest in the Land: New World Epidemics in a Global Perspective.* Albuquerque: University of New Mexico Press, 2003.

Altschuler, Sari. *The Medical Imagination: Literature and Health in the Early United States.* Philadelphia: University of Pennsylvania Press, 2018.

Apel, Thomas. *Feverish Bodies, Enlightened Minds: Science and the Yellow Fever Controversy in the Early American Republic.* Stanford, Calif.: Stanford University Press, 2016.

———. "The Thucydidean Moment: History, Science, and the Yellow-Fever Controversy, 1793–1805." *Journal of the Early Republic* 34, no. 3 (2014): 315–47.

Arikha, Noga. *Passions and Tempers: A History of the Humours.* New York: HarperCollins, 2007.

Arner, Katherine. "Making Yellow Fever American: The Early American Republic, the British Empire and the Geopolitics of Disease in the Atlantic World." *Atlantic Studies* 7, no. 4 (2010): 447–71.

Atwater, Edward C. "The Protracted Labor and Brief Life of a Country Medical School: The Auburn Medical Institution, 1825." *Journal of the History of Medicine and Allied Sciences* 34, no. 3 (1979): 334–52.

Bailyn, Bernard. *The Ideological Origins of the American Revolution*. Cambridge, Mass.: Belknap Press of Harvard University Press, 1967.

Baldwin, Peter. *Contagion and the State in Europe, 1830–1930*. Cambridge: Cambridge University Press, 1999.

Ball, Clara Sue. "The Early History of the Compound Microscope." *Bios* 37, no. 2 (1966): 51–60.

Barcia, Manuel. *The Yellow Demon of Fever: Fighting Disease in the Nineteenth-Century Transatlantic Slave Trade*. New Haven, Conn.: Yale University Press, 2020.

Barnes, David S. "Cargo, 'Infection,' and the Logic of Quarantine in the Nineteenth Century." *Bulletin of the History of Medicine* 88, no. 1 (2014): 75–101.

———. *Lazaretto: How Philadelphia Used an Unpopular Quarantine Based on Disputed Science to Accommodate Immigrants and Prevent Epidemics*. Baltimore: Johns Hopkins University Press, 2023.

Bean, William B. *Walter Reed: A Biography*. Charlottesville: University Press of Virginia, 1982.

———. "Walter Reed and the Ordeal of Human Experiments." *Bulletin of the History of Medicine* 51, no. 1 (1977): 75–92.

Bell, Whitfield J., Jr. *The College of Physicians of Philadelphia: A Bicentennial History*. Canton, Mass.: Science History, 1987.

———. *The Colonial Physician and Other Essays*. New York: Science History, 1975.

———. "The Court Martial of William Shippen, Jr., 1780." *Journal of the History of Medicine and Allied Sciences* 19, no. 3 (1964): 218–38.

———. *John Morgan: Continental Doctor*. Philadelphia: University of Pennsylvania Press, 1965.

Berman, Alex. "The Thomsonian Movement and Its Relation to American Pharmacy and Medicine." *Bulletin of the History of Medicine* 25, no. 5 (1951): 405–28.

———. "The Thomsonian Movement and Its Relation to American Pharmacy and Medicine (Continued)." *Bulletin of the History of Medicine* 25, no. 6 (1951): 519–38.

Bewell, Alan. *Romanticism and Colonial Disease*. Baltimore: Johns Hopkins University Press, 1999.

Blake, John B. "Anatomy." In *The Education of American Physicians: Historical Essays*, edited by Ronald L. Numbers, 29–47. Berkeley: University of California Press, 1980.

———. "The Development of American Anatomy Acts." *Journal of American Medical Education* 30, no. 8 (1955): 431–39.

———. "Yellow Fever in Eighteenth-Century America." *Bulletin of the New York Academy of Medicine* 44 (1968): 673–86.

Bliss, Michael. *The Making of Modern Medicine: Turning Points in the Treatment of Disease*. Chicago: University of Chicago Press, 2011.

Bollet, Alfred J. "Amputations in the Civil War." In *Years of Change and Suffering: Modern Perspectives on Civil War Medicine*, edited by James M. Schmidt and Guy R. Hasegawa, 57–67. Roseville, Minn.: Edenborough Press, 2009.

Bowers, John Z. "The Odyssey of Smallpox Vaccination." *Bulletin of the History of Medicine* 55, no. 1 (1981): 17–33.
Breeden, James O. "Body Snatchers and Anatomy Professors: Medical Education in Nineteenth-Century Virginia." *Virginia Magazine of History and Biography* 83, no. 3 (1975): 321–45.
Breslaw, Elaine G. *Lotions, Potions, Pills, and Magic*. New York: New York University Press, 2012.
Brodsky, Alyn. *Benjamin Rush: Patriot and Physician*. New York: Truman Talley Books, 2004.
Brown, Theodore M. "Medicine in the Shadow of the Principia." *Journal of the History of Ideas* 48, no. 4 (1987): 629–48.
Buerki, Robert A. "The Historical Development of an Ethic for American Pharmacy." *Pharmacy in History* 39, no. 2 (1997): 54–72.
———. "Reception of the Germ Theory of Disease in the *American Journal of Pharmacy*." *Pharmacy in History* 13, no. 4 (1971): 158–68.
Burnham, John C. *Health Care in America: A History*. Baltimore: Johns Hopkins University Press, 2015.
Burrell, Sean, and Geoffrey Gill. "The Liverpool Cholera Epidemic of 1832 and Anatomical Dissection—Medical Mistrust and Civil Unrest." *Journal of the History of Medicine and Allied Sciences* 60, no. 4 (2005): 478–98.
Bynum, W. F., and Roy Porter, eds. *Medical Fringe and Medical Orthodoxy, 1750–1850*. London: Routledge Press, 1987.
Carlson, Eric, and Meribeth Simpson. "Benjamin Rush's Medical Use of the Moral Faculty." *Bulletin of the History of Medicine* 39, no. 1 (1965): 22–33.
Carr, Sara Jensen. *The Topography of Wellness: How Health and Disease Shaped the American Landscape*. Charlottesville: University of Virginia Press, 2021.
Carrigan, Jo Ann. "Privilege, Prejudice, and the Strangers' Disease in Nineteenth-Century New Orleans." *Journal of Southern History* 36, no. 4 (1970): 568–78.
Cassedy, James H. "The Microscope in American Medical Science, 1840–1860." *Isis* 67, no. 1 (1976): 76–97.
Chernin, Eli. "Josiah Clark Nott, Insects and Yellow Fever." *Bulletin of the New York Academy of Medicine* 59, no. 9 (1983): 790–802.
Codell, Carter, K. "The Koch-Pasteur Dispute on Establishing the Cause of Anthrax." *Bulletin of the History of Medicine* 62, no. 1 (1988): 42–57.
Conis, Elena. *Vaccine Nation: America's Changing Relationship with Immunization*. Chicago: University of Chicago Press, 2015.
Cook, Harold, and Timothy Walker. "Circulation of Medicine in the Early Modern Atlantic World." *Social History of Medicine* 26, no. 3 (2013): 337–51.
Cooter, Roger, ed. *Studies in the History of Alternative Medicine*. London: Macmillan, 1988.
Corner, Betsy Copping. *William Shippen, Jr.: Pioneer in American Medical Education, a Biographical Essay*. Philadelphia: American Philosophical Society, 1951.
Cowen, David. "Colonial Laws Pertaining to Pharmacy." *Pharmacy in History* 48, no. 1 (2006): 24–30.
———. "Pharmacists and Physicians: An Uneasy Relationship." *Pharmacy in History* 34, no. 1 (1992): 3–16.

Crosby, Alfred W. "Virgin Soil Epidemics as a Factor in the Aboriginal Depopulation in America." *William and Mary Quarterly*, 3rd series, 33 (1976): 289–99.

D'Elia, Donald. *Benjamin Rush: Philosopher of the Revolution*. Philadelphia: American Philosophical Society, 1974.

———. "Dr. Benjamin Rush and the American Medical Revolution." *Proceedings of the American Philosophical Society* 110, no. 4 (1966): 227–34.

Del Regato, Juan A. "Carlos Juan Finlay (1833–1915)." *Journal of Public Health Policy* 22, no. 1 (2001): 98–104.

Devine, Shauna. *Learning from the Wounded: The Civil War and the Rise of American Medical Science*. Chapel Hill: University of North Carolina Press, 2014.

Dine, Sarah Blank. "Diaries and Doctors: Elizabeth Drinker and Philadelphia Medical Practice, 1760–1818." *Pennsylvania History* 68, no. 4 (2001): 413–34.

Duffy, John. *From Humors to Medical Science: A History of American Medicine*. Champaign: University of Illinois Press, 1993.

———. *The Healers: The Rise of the Medical Establishment*. New York: McGraw-Hill, 1976.

Dykstra, David. "The Medical Profession and Patent and Proprietary Medicines during the Nineteenth Century." *Bulletin of the History of Medicine* 29, no. 5 (1955): 401–19.

Espinosa, Mariola. *Epidemic Invasions: Yellow Fever and the Limits of Cuban Independence, 1878–1930*. Chicago: University of Chicago Press, 2009.

———. "The Question of Racial Immunity to Yellow Fever in History and Historiography." *Social Science History* 38, nos. 3–4 (2014): 437–53.

———. "The Threat from Havana: Southern Public Health, Yellow Fever, and the U.S. Intervention in the Cuban Struggle for Independence, 1878–1898." *Journal of Southern History* 72, no. 3 (2006): 541–68.

Estes, J. Worth. "The Pharmacology of Nineteenth-Century Patent Medicines." *Pharmacy in History* 30, no. 1 (1988): 3–18.

———. "The Shakers and Their Proprietary Medicines." *Bulletin of the History of Medicine* 65, no. 2 (1991): 162–84.

———. "Therapeutic Practice in Colonial New England." In *Medicine in Colonial Massachusetts, 1620–1820*, edited by Philip Cash, Eric H. Christianson, and J. Worth Estes, 289–366. Boston: Colonial Society of Massachusetts, 1980.

Estes, J. Worth, and Billy G. Smith, eds. *A Melancholy Scene of Devastation: The Public Response to the 1793 Philadelphia Yellow Fever Epidemic*. Canton, Mass.: Science History, 1997.

Fenn, Elizabeth A. *Pox Americana: The Great Smallpox Epidemic of 1775–82*. New York: Hill and Wang, 2001.

Fett, Sharla M. *Working Cures: Healing, Health, and Power on Southern Slave Plantations*. Chapel Hill: University of North Carolina Press, 2002.

Fillmore, Susan. "Samuel Thomson and His Effect on the American Health Care System." *Pharmacy in History* 28, no. 4 (1986): 188–91.

Finger, Simon. *The Contagious City: The Politics of Public Health in Early Philadelphia*. Ithaca, N.Y.: Cornell University Press, 2012.

Fink, Michael. T. "Before Yellow Fever and Cuba: Walter Reed in Arizona." *Journal of Arizona History* 42, no. 2 (2001): 181–200.

Flannery, Michael A. "Civil War Pharmacy and Medicine: Comparisons and Contexts." *Pharmacy in History* 46, no. 2 (2004): 71–80.

Foletta, Marshall. *Coming to Terms with Democracy: Federalist Intellectuals and the Shaping of an American Culture.* Charlottesville: University Press of Virginia, 2001.

Foucault, Michel. *The Birth of the Clinic: An Archaeology of Medical Perception.* Translated by A. M. Sheridan Smith. 1963; reprint New York, Tavistock, 1973.

Freemon, Frank. *Gangrene and Glory: Medical Care during the American Civil War.* Champaign: University of Illinois Press, 2001.

Fried, Stephen. *Rush: Revolution, Madness, and the Visionary Doctor Who Became a Founding Father.* New York: Crown, 2018.

Fulton, John F., and Elizabeth H. Thomson. "Benjamin Silliman and the Founding of the Sheffield Scientific School." *American Scientist* 36, no. 1 (1948): 102–10.

Funk, Cary. "Key Findings about Americans' Confidence in Science and Their Views on Scientists' Role in Society." Pew Research Center, 12 February 2020. https://www.pewresearch.org/short-reads/2020/02/12/key-findings-about-americans-confidence-in-science-and-their-views-on-scientists-role-in-society.

———. "Polling Shows Signs of Public Trust in Institutions amid the Pandemic." Pew Research Center, 3 June 2020. https://www.pewresearch.org/science/2020/04/07/polling-shows-signs-of-public-trust-in-institutions-amid-pandemic.

Funk, Cary, Brian Kennedy, and Courtney Johnson. "Trust in Medical Scientists Has Grown in U.S., but Mainly among Democrats." Pew Research Center, 21 May 2020. https://www.pewresearch.org/science/2020/05/21/trust-in-medical-scientists-has-grown-in-u-s-but-mainly-among-democrats.

Gehlbach, Stephen H. *American Plagues: Lessons from Our Battles with Disease.* Lanham, Md.: Rowman and Littlefield, 2016.

Gelfand, Toby. "The Origins of a Modern Concept of Medical Specialization: John Morgan's *Discourse* of 1765." *Bulletin of the History of Medicine* 50, no. 4 (1976): 511–35.

Gilchrist, Michael R. "Disease and Infection in the American Civil War." *American Biology Teacher* 60, no. 4 (1998): 258–62.

A Global Strategy to Eliminate Yellow Fever Epidemics (EYE), 2017–2026. World Health Organization. https://apps.who.int/iris/bitstream/handle/10665/272408/9789241513661-eng.pdf?ua=1.

Goodyear, James. "The Sugar Connection: A New Perspective on the History of Yellow Fever." *Bulletin of the History of Medicine* 52, no. 1 (1978): 5–21.

Gossel, Patricia Peck. "Pasteur, Koch and American Bacteriology." *History and Philosophy of the Life Sciences* 22, no. 1 (2000): 81–100.

Griffenhagen George B. "Early American Drug Containers." *Pharmacy in History* 40, nos. 2–3 (1998): 93–98.

Griffenhagen, George B., and James Harvey Young. "Old English Patent Medicines in America." *Pharmacy in History* 34, no. 4 (1992): 199–229.

Griffith, Sally F. "'A Total Dissolution of the Bonds of Society': Community Death and Regeneration in Mathew Carey's *Short Account of the Malignant Fever.*" In *A Melancholy Scene of Devastation: The Public Response to the 1793 Philadelphia Yellow Fever Epidemic,* edited by J. Worth Estes and Billy G. Smith, 45–59. Philadelphia: Science History, 1997.

Grob, Gerald. *The Deadly Truth: A History of Disease in America.* Cambridge, Mass.: Harvard University Press, 2002.

Gronim, Sara Stidstone. "Imagining Inoculation: Smallpox, the Body, and Social Relations of Healing in the Eighteenth Century." *Bulletin of the History of Medicine* 80, no. 2 (2006): 247–68.

Guerrini, Anita. "Archibald Pitcairne and Newtonian Medicine." *Medical History* 31 no. 1 (1987): 70–83.

Hagenbüchle, Roland. "American Literature and the Nineteenth-Century Crisis in Epistemology: The Example of Charles Brockden Brown." *Early American Literature* 23, no. 2 (1988): 121–51.

Haller, John S. *The History of American Homeopathy: The Academic Years, 1820–1935*. New York: Pharmaceutical Products, 2005.

———. *Medical Protestants: The Eclectics in American Medicine, 1825–1939*. Carbondale: Southern Illinois University Press, 1994.

Halttunen, Karen. *Murder Most Foul: The Killer and the American Gothic Imagination*. Cambridge, Mass.: Harvard University Press, 1998.

Hamilton, Marsha J. "Mercury and Water: Two Civil War Surgeons of the 148th Pennsylvania Volunteers." *Pennsylvania History: A Journal of Mid-Atlantic Studies* 75, no. 4 (2008): 467–504.

Harwood, Robert F., and Maurice T. James. *Entomology in Human and Animal Health*. New York: Macmillan, 1979.

Hasegawa, Guy R. "Southern Resources, Southern Medicines." In *Years of Change and Suffering: Modern Perspectives on Civil War Medicine*, edited by James M. Schmidt and Guy R. Hasegawa, 107–25. Roseville, Minn.: Edenborough Press, 2009.

Hatch, Nathan O. *The Democratization of American Christianity*. New Haven, Conn.: Yale University Press, 1991.

Hedges, William. "Benjamin Rush, Charles Brockden Brown, and the American Plague Year." *Early American Literature* 8, no. 1 (1973): 295–311.

Herschthal, Eric. "Antislavery Science in the Early Republic: The Case of Dr. Benjamin Rush." *Early American Studies* 15, no. 2 (2017): 274–307.

Higby, Gregory J. "Professionalism and the Nineteenth-Century American Pharmacist." *Pharmacy in History* 28, no. 3 (1986): 115–24.

Hogarth, Rana A. *Medicalizing Blackness: Making Racial Difference in the Atlantic World, 1780–1840*. Chapel Hill: University of North Carolina Press, 2017.

Holmes, Chris. "Benjamin Rush and the Yellow Fever." *Bulletin of the History of Medicine* 40, no. 3 (1966): 246–63.

Horsfall, W. F. *Medical Entomology*. New York: Ronald Press, 1962.

Horsman, Reginald. *Josiah Nott of Mobile: Southerner, Physician, and Racial Theorist*. Baton Rouge: Louisiana State University Press, 1987.

———. *Race and Manifest Destiny: The Origins of American Racial Anglo-Saxonism*. Cambridge, Mass.: Harvard University Press, 1981.

Humphreys, Margaret. "Appendix II: Yellow Fever since 1793: History and Historiography." In *A Melancholy Scene of Devastation: The Public Response to the 1793 Philadelphia Yellow Fever Epidemic*, edited by J. Worth Estes and Billy G. Smith, 183–98. Philadelphia: Science History, 1997.

———. *Marrow of Tragedy: The Health Crisis of the American Civil War*. Baltimore: Johns Hopkins University Press, 2013.

———. *Yellow Fever and the South*. New Brunswick, N.J.: Rutgers University Press, 1992.
Johnson, Victoria. *American Eden: David Hosack, Botany, and Medicine in the Garden of the Early Republic*. New York: Norton, 2018.
Johnston, Katherine. *The Nature of Slavery: Environment and Plantation Labor in the Anglo-Atlantic World*. New York: Oxford University Press, 2022.
Jones, Richard. *Mosquito*. London: Reaktion Books, 2012.
Kelly, Catherine. "'Not from the College, but Through the Public and the Legislature': Charles Maclean and the Relocation of Medical Debate in the Early Nineteenth Century." *Bulletin of the History of Medicine* 82, no. 3 (2008): 545–69.
Kiechle, Melanie A. *Smell Detectives: An Olfactory History of Nineteenth-Century America*. Seattle: University of Washington Press, 2017.
King, Lester S. "Dr. Koch's Postulates." *Journal of the History of Medicine and Allied Sciences* 7, no. 4 (1952): 350–61.
———. *Transformations in American Medicine: From Benjamin Rush to William Osler*. Baltimore: Johns Hopkins University Press, 1992.
Kiple, Kenneth, and Virginia Kiple. "Black Yellow Fever Immunities, Innate and Acquired, as Revealed in the American South." *Social Science History* 1, no. 4 (1977): 419–36.
Klaw, Spencer. "Belly My Grizzle." *American Heritage* 28, no. 4 (1977): 96–102.
Klepp, Susan E. "'How Many Precious Souls Are Fled': The Magnitude of the 1793 Yellow Fever Epidemic." In *A Melancholy Scene of Devastation: The Public Response to the 1793 Philadelphia Yellow Fever Epidemic*, edited by J. Worth Estes and Billy G. Smith, 163–82. Philadelphia: Science History, 1997.
Kopperman, Paul. "'Venerate the Lancet': Benjamin Rush's Yellow Fever Therapy in Context." *Bulletin of the History of Medicine* 78, no. 3 (2004): 539–74.
Kornfield, Eve. "Crisis in the Capital: The Cultural Significance of Philadelphia's Great Yellow Fever Epidemic." *Pennsylvania History: A Journal of Mid-Atlantic Studies* 51, no. 3 (1984): 189–205.
Lapsansky, Philip. "'Abigail, a Negress': The Role and the Legacy of African Americans in the Yellow Fever Epidemic." In *A Melancholy Scene of Devastation: The Public Response to the 1793 Philadelphia Yellow Fever Epidemic*, edited by J. Worth Estes and Billy G. Smith, 61–78. Philadelphia: Science History, 1997.
Lawrence, C. J. "William Buchan: Medicine Laid Open." *Medical History* 19, no. 1 (1975): 20–35.
Leavitt, Judith Walzer. "'Science' Enters the Birthing Room: Obstetrics in America since the Eighteenth Century." *Journal of American History* 70, no. 2 (1983): 281–304.
———. "Under the Shadow of Maternity: American Women's Responses to Death and Debility Fears in Nineteenth-Century Childbirth." *Feminist Studies* 12, no. 1 (1986): 129–54.
Levine, Paul. "The American Novel Begins." *American Scholar* 35, no. 1 (1965): 134–48.
Longo, Lawrence D. "Obstetrics and Gynecology." In *The Education of American Physicians: Historical Essays*, edited by Ronald L. Numbers, 205–25. Berkeley: University of California Press, 1980.
Loudin, Irvine. "The Vile Race of Quacks with Which This Country Is Infested." In *Medical Fringe and Medical Orthodoxy, 1750–1850*, edited by W. F. Bynum and Roy Porter, 106–28. London: Routledge Press, 1987.

Louis, Elan Daniel. "William Shippen's Unsuccessful Attempt to Establish the First 'School for Physick' in the American Colonies in 1762." *Journal of the History of Medicine and Allied Sciences* 44, no. 2 (1989): 218–39.

Ludmerer, Kenneth M. *Learning to Heal: The Development of American Medical Education.* New York: Basic Books, 1985.

Mark, Catherine, and José G. Rigan-Pérez. "The World's First Immunization Campaign: The Spanish Smallpox Vaccine Expedition, 1803–13." *Bulletin of the History of Medicine* 83, no. 1 (2009): 63–94.

Maulitz, Russell. "Pathology." In *The Education of American Physicians: Historical Essays*, edited by Ronald L. Numbers, 29–47. Berkeley: University of California Press, 1980.

May, Henry. *The Enlightenment in America.* Oxford: Oxford University Press, 1976.

McMahon, Michael. "Beyond Therapeutics: Technology and the Question of Public Health in Late Eighteenth-Century Philadelphia." In *A Melancholy Scene of Devastation: The Public Response to the 1793 Philadelphia Yellow Fever Epidemic*, edited by J. Worth Estes and Billy G. Smith, 97–117. Philadelphia: Science History, 1997.

McNeill, J. R. *Mosquito Empires: Ecology and War in the Greater Caribbean, 1620–1914.* New York: Cambridge University Press, 2010.

Middleton, William. "Felix Pascalis-Ouvière and the Yellow Fever Epidemic of 1797." *Bulletin of the History of Medicine* 38, no. 6 (1964): 497–515.

Mukharji, Projit Bihari. "The 'Cholera Cloud' in the Nineteenth-Century 'British World': History of an Object-without-an-Essence." *Bulletin of the History of Medicine* 86, no. 3 (2012): 303–32.

Murphy, Lamar Riley. *Enter the Physician: The Transformation of Domestic Medicine, 1760–1860.* Tuscaloosa: University of Alabama Press, 1991.

Mutschler, Ben. *The Province of Affliction: Illness and the Making of Early New England.* Chicago: University of Chicago Press, 2020.

Naramore, Sara. *Benjamin Rush, Civic Health, and Human Illness in the Early American Republic.* Rochester, N.Y.: University of Rochester Press, 2023.

Nord, David Paul. "Readership as Citizenship in Late-Eighteenth-Century Philadelphia." In *A Melancholy Scene of Devastation: The Public Response to the 1793 Philadelphia Yellow Fever Epidemic*, edited by J. Worth Estes and Billy G. Smith, 19–44. Philadelphia: Science History, 1997.

Nuland, Sherwin B. *The Doctors' Plague: Germs, Childbed Fever, and the Strange Story of Ignác Semmelweiss.* New York: Norton, 2000.

Numbers, Ronald L., ed. *The Education of American Physicians: Historical Essays.* Berkeley: University of California Press, 1980.

Olivarius, Kathryn. *Necropolis: Disease, Power, and Capitalism in the Cotton Kingdom.* Cambridge, Mass.: Belknap Press of Harvard University Press, 2022.

Olton, Charles. "Philadelphia's First Environmental Class." *Pennsylvania Magazine of History and Biography* 98, no. 1 (1974): 90–100.

Packard, Randall M. "'Break-Bone' Fever in Philadelphia, 1780: Reflections on the History of Disease." *Bulletin of the History of Medicine* 90, no. 2 (2016): 193–221.

Parascandola, John. "The Emergence of Pharmaceutical Science." *Pharmacy in History* 37, no. 2 (1995): 68–75.

Parsons, Gail Pat. "Puerperal Fever, Anticontagionists, and Miasmatic Infection, 1840–1860: Toward a New History of Puerperal Fever in Antebellum America." *Journal of the History of Medicine and Allied Sciences* 52, no. 4 (1997): 424–52.
Peckham, C. H. "A Brief History of Puerperal Infection." *Bulletin of the Institute of the History of Medicine* 3, no. 3 (1935): 187–212.
Peller, Sigismund. "Walter Reed, C. Finlay, and Their Predecessors around 1800." *Bulletin of the History of Medicine* 33, no. 3 (1959): 195–211.
Peterson, Merrill D. *Thomas Jefferson and the New Nation*. New York: Oxford University Press, 1970.
Pierce, John, and Jim Writer. *Yellow Jack: How Yellow Fever Ravaged America and Walter Reed Discovered Its Deadly Secrets*. Hoboken, N.J.: Wiley, 2005.
Ponce, Rachel N. "'They Increase in Beauty and Elegance': Transforming Cadavers and the Epistemology of Dissection in Early Nineteenth-Century American Medical Education." *Journal of the History of Medicine and Allied Sciences* 68, no. 3 (2013): 331–76.
Porter, Roy. "Before the Fringe: 'Quackery' and the Eighteenth-Century Medical Market." In *Studies in the History of Alternative Medicine*, edited by Roger Cooter, 1–27. London: Macmillan, 1988.
———. "The Patient in England, c. 1660–c. 1800." In *Medicine in Society: Historical Essays*, edited by Andrew Wear, 91–118. Cambridge: Cambridge University Press, 1992.
Porter, Roy, and Dorothy Porter. "The Rise of the English Drug Industry: The Role of Thomas Corbyn." *Medical History* 33 (1989): 277–95.
Powell, J. H. *Bring Out Your Dead: The Great Plague of Yellow Fever in Philadelphia in 1793*. Philadelphia: University of Pennsylvania Press, 1949.
Rogers, Naomi. "The Proper Place of Homeopathy: Hahnemann Medical College and Hospital in an Age of Scientific Medicine." *Pennsylvania Magazine of History and Biography* 108, no. 2 (1984): 179–201.
Rosenberg, Charles. *The Cholera Years: The United States in 1832, 1849, and 1866*. Chicago: University of Chicago Press, 1962.
———. "The Therapeutic Revolution: Medicine, Meaning, and Social Change in Nineteenth-Century America." In *The Therapeutic Revolution: Essays in the Social History of American Medicine*, edited by Morris J. Vogel and Charles E. Rosenberg, 3–26. Philadelphia: University of Pennsylvania Press, 1979.
Rosner, Lisa. "Thistle on the Delaware: Edinburgh's Medical Education and Philadelphia Practice, 1800–1825." *Social History of Medicine* 5, no. 1 (1992): 19–42.
Rossiter, Margaret W. "Benjamin Silliman and the Lowell Institute: The Popularization of Science in Nineteenth-Century America." *New England Quarterly* 44, no. 4 (1971): 602–26.
Rothstein, William G. *American Physicians in the Nineteenth Century: From Sects to Science*. Baltimore: Johns Hopkins University Press, 1985.
Ruestow, Edward G. *The Microscope in the Dutch Republic: The Shaping of Discovery*. Cambridge: Cambridge University Press, 1995.
Rusnock, Andrea. "Catching Cowpox: The Early Spread of Smallpox Vaccination, 1798–1810." *Bulletin of the History of Medicine* 83, no. 1 (2009): 17–36.
Rutkow, Ira. *Seeking the Cure: A History of Medicine in America*. New York: Scribner, 2010.

Sappol, Michael. *A Traffic of Dead Bodies: Anatomy and Embodied Social Identity in Nineteenth-Century America*. Princeton, N.J.: Princeton University Press, 2002.

Savitt, Todd L. *Medicine and Slavery: The Diseases and Health Care of Blacks in Antebellum Virginia*. Urbana: University of Illinois Press, 1978.

———. "The Use of Blacks for Medical Experimentation and Demonstration in the Old South." *Journal of Southern History* 48, no. 3 (1982): 331–48.

Schultz, Myron G. "Photo Quiz—Henry Rose Carter." *Emerging Infectious Diseases* 15, no. 10 (2009): 1682–84.

Service, R. W. "A Short History of Early Medical Entomology." *Journal of Medical Entomology* 14, no. 6 (1978): 603–26.

Shryock, Richard Harrison. "The Fielding H. Garrison Lecture: The Medical Reputation of Benjamin Rush: Contrasts over Two Centuries." *Bulletin of the History of Medicine* 45, no. 6 (1971): 507–52.

———. "A Medical Perspective on the Civil War." *American Quarterly* 14, no. 2 (1962): 161–73.

Smith, Billy G. *Ship of Death: A Voyage That Changed the Atlantic World*. New Haven, Conn.: Yale University Press, 2013.

Smith, George F. *The Man Who Saved the World from Smallpox: Doctor Edward Jenner*. New York: iUniverse, 2004.

Smith, Mark. "Andrew Brown's 'Earnest Endeavor': The *Federal Gazette*'s Role in Philadelphia's Yellow Fever Epidemic of 1793." *Pennsylvania Magazine of History and Biography* 120, no. 4 (1996): 321–42.

Sonnedecker, Glenn. "The Founding Period of the U.S. Pharmacopeia: II. A National Movement Emerges." *Pharmacy in History* 36, no. 1 (1994): 3–25.

———. "The Founding Period of the U. S. Pharmacopeia: III. The First Edition." *Pharmacy in History* 36, no. 3 (1994): 103–22.

Starr, Paul. *The Transformation of American Medicine: The Rise of a Sovereign Profession and the Making of a Vast Industry*. New York: Basic Books, 1982.

Stepan, Nancy. "The Interplay between Socio-Economic Factors and Medical Science: Yellow Fever Research, Cuba and the United States." *Social Studies of Science* 8, no. 4 (1978): 397–423.

Stover, Kate F., and Ara Der Marderosian. "The Philadelphia College of Pharmacy and Science Preserves Its History." *Pharmacy in History* 38, no. 1 (1996): 29–33.

Stroud, Patricia Tyson. *Thomas Say: New World Naturalist*. Philadelphia: University of Pennsylvania Press, 1992.

Sullivan, Robert B. "Sanguine Practices: A Historical and Historiographic Reconsideration of Heroic Therapy in the Age of Rush." *Bulletin of the History of Medicine* 68, no. 2 (1994): 211–34.

Unger, Harlow Giles. *Dr. Benjamin Rush: The Founding Father Who Healed a Wounded Nation*. New York: Da Capo Press, 2018.

Valenčius, Conevery Bolton. *The Health of the Country: How American Settlers Understood Themselves and Their Land*. New York: Basic Books, 2002.

Viets, Henry R. "Oliver Wendell Holmes, Physician." *American Scholar* 3, no. 1 (1934): 4–11.

Vogel, Morris J., and Charles E. Rosenberg, eds. *The Therapeutic Revolution: Essays in the Social History of American Medicine*. Philadelphia: University of Pennsylvania Press, 1979.

Waring, Joseph Ioor. "The Influence of Benjamin Rush on the Practice of Bleeding in South Carolina." *Bulletin of the History of Medicine* 35, no. 3 (1961): 230–37.
Warner, John Harley. *Against the Spirit of the System: The French Impulse in Nineteenth-Century American Medicine.* Baltimore: Johns Hopkins University Press, 1998.
———. *The Therapeutic Perspective: Medical Practice, Knowledge, and Identity in America, 1820–1885.* Cambridge, Mass.: Harvard University Press, 1986.
Waterman, Bryan. *Republic of Intellect: The Friendly Club of New York City and the Making of American Literature.* Baltimore: Johns Hopkins University Press, 2007.
Wear, Andrew, ed. *Medicine in Society: Historical Essays.* Cambridge: Cambridge University Press, 1992.
Wehrman, Andrew. *The Contagion of Liberty: The Politics of Smallpox in the American Revolution.* Baltimore: Johns Hopkins University Press, 2022.
———. "The Siege of 'Castle Pox': A Medical Revolution in Marblehead, Massachusetts, 1764–77." *New England Quarterly* 82, no. 3 (2009): 385–429.
Weiner, Dora B., and Michael J. Sauter. "The City of Paris and the Rise of Clinical Medicine." *Osiris* 18 (2003): 23–42.
Will, Thomas. "Liberalism, Republicanism, and Philadelphia's Black Elite in the Early Republic: The Social Thought of Absalom Jones and Richard Allen." *Pennsylvania History* 69, no. 4 (2002): 558–76.
Williams, William H. "The 'Industrious Poor' and the Founding of the Pennsylvania Hospital." *Pennsylvania Magazine of History and Biography* 97, no. 4 (1973): 431–43.
Willoughby, Christopher. *Masters of Health: Racial Science and Slavery in U.S. Medical Schools.* Chapel Hill: University of North Carolina Press, 2022.
Wilson, Catherine. *The Invisible World: Early Modern Philosophy and the Invention of the Microscope.* Princeton, N.J.: Princeton University Press, 1995.
Wilson, Renate. "Trading in Drugs through Philadelphia in the Eighteenth Century: A Transatlantic Enterprise." *Social History of Medicine* 26, no. 3 (2013): 352–63.
Wilson, Renate, and Woodrow J. Savacool. "The Theory and Practice of Pharmacy in Pennsylvania: Observations on Two Colonial Country Doctors." *Pennsylvania History: A Journal of Mid-Atlantic Studies* 68, no. 1 (2001): 31–65.
Woodruff, Lorande Loss. "The Advent of the Microscope at Yale College." *American Scientist* 31, no. 3 (1943): 241–45.

INDEX

Adams, John, 28, 53
Adams, Samuel, 28, 61
Aedes aegypti, 21. *See also* mosquitos
Allen, Richard, 17, 87, 230n40
American Entomology. See Say, Thomas
American Journal of Science, 138–39
American Medical Association, 151–52, 199
American Pharmaceutical Association, 152
Andry, Nicholas, 174
anesthetics: in Civil War, 202–3; development of, 202
animalcular theories: ancient and medieval, 170–71; early modern, 177–83; and Nott, 13, 160–62, 169–70, 180–81
Apel, Thomas, 39
apothecaries: and advertising, 64, 65; in Britain, 66; and "druggists," 65–66; and founding of Philadelphia College of Pharmacy, 141–42; and the growing drug market, 62; within Morgan's reform vision, 64, 67. *See also* pharmacists
Aristotle, 174
Arthur Mervyn, 131–33
Audubon, James, 182

Bailyn, Bernard, 39
Ball's Wharf, 16, 27

Balmis, Francisco Javier de, 104
Bard, Samuel, 47
bark. *See* quinine
Bartlett, Elisha, 5, 38
Barton, Benjamin Smith, 97
Beauperthuy, Louis-Daniel, 212
Beguerie, J. M., 96
Beugnot, J. F., 167
Black bodies: beliefs on physiological difference, 184–89; and disease immunity, 8, 17, 22–24, 165–66, 184; medical school use of, 186, 196; Nott on, 184, 187–91; and proslavery apologetic, 23, 185; Rush on, 184–85
Black people: as caregivers during epidemic, 8, 17, 23, 87, 184; criticism of during epidemic and response to, 8, 230n40; disease immunity, 8, 17, 23–24, 165–66, 184; and French vaccination campaign, 108; as plantation healers, 100; as plantation slaves, 23, 165, 186; revolution in Saint-Domingue, 212; Rush on slavery as depressive stimulus, 185; whites on miscegenation, 191
bleeding. *See* depletion therapy
Boerhaave, Herman, 29, 43
Bonaparte, Napoleon, 212
Bond, Thomas, Jr., 57

Bond, Thomas, Sr., 48, 51, 57
Bonomo, Giovanni, 170
Bradford, William, 111
Bradley, Richard, 178–79. *See also* animalcular theories
Brief History of Epidemic and Pestilential Diseases, 125. *See also* Webster, Noah
Brown, Charles Brockden, 90, 131–33
Brown, John, 30, 43
Brown, Samuel, 95–96, 140
Buchan, William, 63
Buel, William, 93. *See also* Smith, Elihu Hubbard
Buffon, Comte de, 6, 182
Bush Hill, 17

Caldwell, Charles, 126, 187
Calomel, 4, 16, 27, 35, 37, 40, 41, 64, 77, 98, 113, 115, 119, 150, 202. *See also* depletion therapy
Carey, Mathew, 131–32
Carlos IV, King of Spain, 104
Carpenter, George W., 141
Carter, Henry Rose, 215–16
Cathrall, Isaac, 82, 156–57, 217
Centennial Exposition, Philadelphia, 209
Channing, Henry, 140
chemistry, 28, 48, 50, 95, 139–41, 146, 155, 158, 195
Chervin, Nicolas, 120
childbed fever. *See* puerperal fever
Chisholm, Colin, 79
cholera, 5; American epidemic, 123–24; Canadian epidemic, 121–24; contagiousness of, 120; diagnostic and therapeutic pessimism, 124–26; European preventive measures and resistance to, 119–20, 233n8; "gothic" response in US, 126–30; mobility and virulence, 118; "morbus" versus "Asiatic" or "spasmodic," 118

Church, Benjamin, 51
Church, John, 108
Civil War, 5, 13; anesthetics, 202–3; army medical museum, 206–7; and depletion therapy, 202; fears of wartime epidemic, 208; medical reform efforts, including nursing, 204–7; mortality, 203, 206; understanding of infection, 203
Clarkson, Matthew, 15, 16, 71
Cobbett, William, 86, 88
College of Philadelphia, 46, 48, 68, 69, 92; and Morgan's medical school proposal, 49–50, 53; and Rush, 28; and Elihu Smith, 92
College of Physicians (of Philadelphia), 4, 15, 18, 39, 69–70, 71, 75, 95
contagionism: and cholera, 119–20, 123; and puerperal fever, 135, 136; and yellow fever, 73, 79, 80, 82–84, 85, 89, 167, 214. *See also* Currie, William
Continental Army, medical care within, 51–57. *See also* Morgan, John; Rush, Benjamin; Shippen, William, Jr.
Cooke, T. A., 167, 168
Cooper, Thomas, 184
COVID-19, 1–2, 10
cowpox. *See* Jenner, Edward
Coxe, John Redman, 84, 87–88, 98, 108
Crawford, John, 179–80. *See also* animalcular theories
Cuba: revolution in, 212, 213; as source of yellow fever, 212–13; yellow fever research in, 213–16. *See also* Reed, Walter
Cullen, William, 28, 43, 224n7
Currie, William, 69, 73–75, 79–82, 84, 87, 88, 96, 97. *See also* contagionism
Curtis, Alva, 151

Danielson, L., 98
Davaine, Casimir, 210

Davidson, George, 95
de Graaf, Regnier, 175
De mulierum morbis, 134
dengue fever, 2
depletion therapy, 3–4; in child birthing, 100; during Civil War, 202; criticism of Rush's use, 5, 43, 73, 75, 97, 98; Deveze on, 77; lay self-bleeding, 99; in *Medical Repository*, 90–91, 94; Nassy on, 78; perceived effectiveness of, 114–15; popularity of, 111, 112–15; Rush's use of, 5, 16, 27, 35–36, 38, 40–42, 112; slave healers use of, 100; in the South, 167; Thomson on, 147, 150
Descartes, René, 31
Deveze, Jean, 77–78, 83
Dewees, William, 100–101, 109–10
Dimsdale, Thomas, 60
dissection, 196; anatomy acts regarding, 198; cultural and legal opposition to, 196–97; educative value of, 197; as student ritual, 197–98
Dix, Dorothea, 204
Drinker, Elizabeth, 17
Duer, William, 53, 54
Dunlap, John, 59
Dunlap, William, 91

Eakins, Thomas, 209–10
Ebola, 1
Echo, 92. *See also* Smith, Elihu Hubbard
eclecticism, 158
effluvia. *See* miasma
Ehrenberg, Christian, 169, 181
emboîtement, 175. *See also* preformation
epidemics, puerperal fever, 134–35. *See also* cholera; Philadelphia epidemic of 1793; yellow fever, epidemics
epigenesis, 174–75

Fenner, E. D., 166
Fenno, John, Jr., 86
Ffirth, Stubbins, 83
Finlay, Juan Carlos, 211–12, 214–15
Fothergill, John, 46–47
Foulke, John, 69
Franklin, Benjamin, 51
Freedmen's Bureau, 193

Galen, 3, 141, 205
Gardiner, William H., 133
Girard, Stephen, 17
Goldson, William, 102, 107; rebutted, 107–8
Gordon, Alexander of Aberdeen, 135
gothic: in American medical culture, 126–31; themes in literature, 127–28, 131–33
Graham, Sylvester, 157
Gram, Hans, 154
Greene, Nathanael, 53, 54
Griffitts, Samuel, 114
Gross, Samuel, 209–10
Gross Clinic, The (Eakins), 210

Hahnemann, Samuel. *See* homeopathy
Haiti. *See* Saint-Domingue, Haiti
Hamilton, Alfred, 205
Hammond, William, 202, 205, 206–7
Hankey (ship), 79–80
Hardie, James, 79–80
Harris, Thaddeus William, 181
Harris, Tudor, 97
Hartsoeker, Nicolaas, 175–77
Harvey, William, 174–75
Hauptmann, August, 171
Henry, William, 138
heroic therapy. *See* depletion therapy
Hippocrates, 126, 134
Holland, Sir Henry, 169, 179. *See also* animalcular theories

Holmes, Oliver Wendell: on homeopathy, 155; on puerperal fever, 135; on Rush, 115–16
homeopathy, 12, 154–57; critique of, 155; laws of similars and minimum dose, 154–55; schism within, 157
Hooke, Robert, 171–73, 177
Hopkinson, Francis, 58
Hort, W. P., 166
Hosack, Alexander, 95
humoral theory, 3, 148, 153, 170, 216
Hunter, George, 114
Hunter, John, 46, 48, 50, 53, 103
Hunter, William, 50
Hutchinson, James, 57
hydropathy, 157

indigenous medicine, 6–7
inoculation, 59–62; during American Revolution, 105–6; commercial opportunities, 61–62; opposition to, 60–61
"irregular" practitioners, 117, 137–38, 157–58, 159. *See also* homeopathy; Thomson, Samuel

Janssen, Hans and Sacharias, 171
Jefferson, Thomas: and America's scientific potential, 6–7; and Jennerian vaccination, 105; rebuts de Buffon, 6, 182
Jenner, Edward, 102–5. *See also* smallpox
Jones, Absalom, 17, 87, 230n40
Journal of the Philadelphia College of Pharmacy, 142. *See also* pharmacists

Koch, Robert, 2, 158, 159, 209–11, 216
Kuhn, Adam, 4, 42, 73–75, 84

Latrobe, Benjamin, 162
Lavoisier, Antoine-Laurent, 140. *See also* chemistry

law of minimum dose. *See* homeopathy
law of similars. *See* homeopathy
Lazear, Jesse, 215
Le Conte, John, 182
Lee, Richard Henry, 51
Leibniz, Gottfried Wilhelm, 31
LeMaigre, Catherine, 15
Letterman, Jonathan, 204
Lewis, J. Hampden, 167
Lewis, P. H., 166
Lining, John, 23, 184
Linnaeus, Carl, 169
Lister, Joseph, 209, 210
Lobelia. *See* Thomsonianism
Long, Stephen, 182
Louis, Pierre Charles Alexander, 135

Mackenzie, Colin, 48
Maclean, Charles, 120
Madison, James, 39
malaria, 62, 138, 154, 203, 212, 213, 214
Malpighi, Marcello, 177
Mann, E., 98
Mann, James, 98
Manson, Patrick, 212
Marblehead riots, 61
Massie, J. C., 168
Mather, Cotton, 60
Medical and Agricultural Register, 97–98
Medical and Surgical History of the War of the Rebellion, 207
medical education: Americans studying in Europe, 200–202; European and American medical education compared, 199–201, 240n15; lax admission standards and curricula, 195–96; and microscopes, 158, 173, 195; nineteenth century increase in medical schools, 194; obstetrics training, 198; and pathology, 195, 216; reform

proposals, including AMA, 198–99. *See also* dissection
medical marketplace: emergence of "druggist," 65–66; increased consumer/patient choices, and inoculation, 62–63; new opportunities for physicians, 59–62; physician-lay tension, 66–69; role of advertising, 64–67
Medical Repository, 11–12, 38, 90–91; on Rush and depletion therapy, 94–96, 110, 139–40
Meigs, Charles, 135–36
Meredith, Margaret, 114
miasma: in *Arthur Mervyn*, 132; as cause of disease generally, 9, 26, 40, 95–96, 98, 106, 111–12, 116, 117, 138–40, 164, 166, 195; and cholera, 119–20; and the Civil War, 203, 206, 207, 208; Currie on, 73, 79, 81; Nott on, 160, 180, 192; public embrace of miasmatic theory, 110–12, 219; and puerperal fever, 136; Rush on, 26, 34, 40; Elihu Smith on, 94; sources of, 26, 78, 94, 95, 98, 140, 164; in the South, 166–69; Webster on, 126; and yellow fever, 26, 34, 37, 77, 78, 79, 94–96, 97, 166–67, 212
Micrographia. *See* Hooke, Robert
microscope: in America, 173; difficulty in use, 173–74; discovery of, 171; and insects, 171–72; and spermatozoa, 174–77
Mifflin, Thomas, 84, 85
Miller, Edward, 96
Minié, Claude-Étienne, 204
Mitchell, John, 37, 41
Mitchell, Samuel, 96, 139–40, 142
Mobile, Alabama, yellow fever epidemics, 161–62, 164
Moderatus, Lucius Junius, 170
Montreal, smallpox epidemic, 10
Morgagni, Giovanni Battista, 49

Morgan, John: attacks on Shippen, 52–53, 55; as director general and chief physician of Continental Army, 51–52; education, 46–47, 48, 50; European tour, 48–49; medical school proposal, 47, 49–51; and professional reform, 66–67, 68
mortality: cholera, 129; Civil War, 203, 204, 206; smallpox, 102, 106, 108. *See also* yellow fever, mortality
Morton, Samuel George, 187–90
Morton, William Thomas Green, 202
mosquitos, 2, 13, 72, 80, 229n3; behavior of, 21; and Finlay, 212; habitat expansion in Latin America, 21; northern versus southern habitats in US, 164–65; and Nott, 170; and Reed, 214–16
Moss, Henry, 185
Murray, Alfred, 162

Nassy, David de Isaac Cohen, 78
New Orleans, and yellow fever, 164–66, 208
New Orleans Medical and Surgical Journal, 166–69
Nott, Josiah Clark, 12–13, 159, 160–62; animalcular theories, 169–70, 183; death of children, 160–62; influence of Thomas Cooper, 184; on miscegenation, 191–92, 193; racial theories, 184–85, 187–92; religious iconoclasm, 190

Owen, Robert, 183

Pascalis-Ouvière, Felix, 78–79
Pasteur, Louis, 2, 210
Patent (or proprietary) medicines, 62–67; advertising of, 64–67; pharmacists' and physicians' response to, 64, 144–46, 151–53
Peale, Charles Willson, 29, 88
Penn, Thomas, 50
Pennington, John, 74–75

Pennsylvania Packet, 55–58
Peters, Richard, 49
pharmacists, 12, 141–47; and chemistry, 141–42, 158; and *The Pharmacopeia of the United States*, 142–44, 158–59; Philadelphia College of Pharmacy and journal, 141–42, 158; response to patent/proprietary medicines, 144–47; and Thomsonianism, 146–47, 151, 152–53. *See also* apothecaries
Pharmacopeia of the United States of America, The: criticism of, 143–44; drafting of, 142–43
Philadelphia: Ball's Wharf, 15–16; College of Pharmacy, 141–42; College of Physicians, 4, 15, 18, 39, 69–70, 71, 75, 95; medical commission on cholera, 121–22, 124–26; medical establishment, divisions within, 18, 38–40, 45–59, 60, 73–75, 79, 87; medical marketplace, 59, 62–68; medical school and hospital, 3, 28, 29–30, 45, 47–51, 53, 57, 59, 68–69; public health measures, 7–8, 18, 45, 163, 164; smallpox inoculation, 59–60, 61–62; yellow fever epidemics after 1793, 84–89
Philadelphia epidemic of 1793, 3–5, 15; ad hoc committees to address, 17; appeals to Black community, 17, 87; Currie and Kuhn on, 73–75; dispute among physicians, 73–75; lay analysis and remedies, 27, 72, 75–76, 88–89; modernizing consequences of, 7–8; mortality, 16, 17–18, 28; post-epidemic medical studies, 77–79, 82–83; post-epidemic sanitation campaigns, 162–64; research on black vomit, 82–83; Rush on, 16, 34–36, 37, 41–42, 74–75
Philadelphia Medical and Physical Journal, 97
Philadelphia Medical Museum, 98–99, 107–9
Pollender, Aloys, 210

polygenesis, 184, 187–92
Porcupine's Gazette. *See* Cobbett, William
Porter, John, 75
Powell, J. H., 38–39, 43
preformation, 175–77
puerperal fever: clusters in the US, 134–35; Holmes on, 135; Meigs on, 135–36; symptoms and explanations, 134
purging. *See* depletion therapy
putrefaction. *See* miasma

quarantines: during cholera epidemic, 120, 123, 129, 139; and Philadelphia, 84, 97, 163–64
quinine (bark), 36, 42, 62, 64, 73, 75, 114, 115, 141, 154, 203

Rafinesque, Samuel, 158
Ramsey, David, 43
Redman, John, 28, 53
Reed, Walter, 214–16
Rhinelander, J. R., 123–24
Riddell, John L., 180. *See also* animalcular theories
Royal College of Physicians, 18, 45, 46, 49, 69, 120
Royal Jennerian Society, 108
Royal Society (of London), 49, 103
Rush, Benjamin, 4, 11, 13; attacked by Cobbett and Fenno, 86–88; criticism of Shippen, 54–55, 56–57; critique of, 38–40, 73–75, 79, 87; education, 28, 53; epidemic explained, treatment recommended, 16, 34–36, 37, 41–42; Holmes on, 115–16; on indigenous medicines, 6–7; medical practice, 28, 61; *Medical Repository* on, 90–91, 94–96; medical theories, 30–34, 40–42; popularity of Rush and his therapeutics, 111–15; as professor, 29–30, 43; on relationship between physicians

and patients, 67–68; as surgeon general of the Continental Army for the middle states, 29, 53–54; on Webster's "atmospheric" theories, 126

Rush, Julia, 36, 37

Ruston, Thomas, 42

Saint-Domingue, Haiti, 15, 16, 79, 80

Sanarelli, Giuseppe, 214

sanitation campaigns: in Cuba, 213; logic behind, 111, 163; in Philadelphia, 7–8, 18, 163, 164; in the South, 164, 165, 169, 208

SARS, 1

Say, Thomas, 181–84

scarlatina (scarlet fever), 139

self-mastery, 9, 11, 115, 116, 219

septon, 139–40

Shakespeare, Edward, 216

Shattuck, George, 97

Shippen, William, Jr.: attacked in the press, 55–57; court martial of, 55; education, 46–48; intellectual character, 50, 226n10; medical position with Continental Army, 52; medical school proposal, 48; resignation from military medical corps, 58

Shryock, Richard Harrison, 205

Silliman, Benjamin, 138–40

smallpox: inoculation, 59–62; Jenner and vaccination, 102–9; Montreal epidemic, 10; vaccination campaigns, imperial, 104. *See also* inoculation

Smith, Daniel, 142

Smith, Elias, 149, 150–51

Smith, Elihu Hubbard, 12, 90–95, 110, 116, 132; diary, 92–93; education and early career, 91–92; launches *Medical Repository*, 93–95; promotion of Rush's medical ideas, 94–95; use of tobacco in child birthing, 100

Smith, Samuel, 99

Smith, Southwood, 138

Smith, Thomas, 97

Snow, John, 118

Spanish American War: post-war sanitation efforts, 216; US yellow fever research, 213–16; yellow fever as reason for US entry, 212–13

Spaulding, Lyman, 142

Spence, John, 108

Spencer Microscope, 173–74

State Island inspection station, 163

Sternberg, George, 213–14, 216

Stevens, Edward, 36, 74

stimuli: body's dependence on, 30; "excitability," 31, 224n12; and health and illness, 33; physician's role in regulating, 33–34, 40–41; sources of, 30–31; sthenic versus asthenic fevers, 33; and yellow fever epidemic, 34

Sutton, Robert, 60; smallpox inoculation, 59–62

Sydenham, Thomas, 74, 126

Thomson, Samuel: life and experience with conventional medicine, 147; as practitioner, 147–48. *See also* Thomsonianism

Thomsonianism, 12, 146–54; critique of conventional medicine, 149–50; demographic and regional concentration, 153–54; distribution network, 148–49; and Jacksonian American, 149; response of pharmacists and regular physicians, 151–53; schism within, 151; therapeutics, 148, 150. *See also* Thomson, Samuel

Thurber, W. J., 168

Tilton, James, 56, 86

Tinicum Island Lazaretto/quarantine station, 163–64

Troth, Henry, 144, 152

University of Michigan, 195
University of Pennsylvania, 57, 68, 79; introduces master's degree in pharmacy, 141; medical school faculty, 59; merger with College of Philadelphia, 29; and Rush, 29–30, 59
US Centers for Disease Control, 1–2
Ussher, James, 190
US Yellow Fever Commission, 212

Van Leeuwenhoek, Antonie, 171–72, 174
Varro, Marcus Terentius, 170
Vaughan, John, 102
venesection. *See* depletion therapy

Washington, George, 15
Waterhouse, Benjamin, 105
Watkins, T., 101
Webster, Noah, 91, 125–26
Welch, William Henry, 216
Wesley, John, 63
Wheaton, L., 96
Williams, William G., 166
Wistar, Caspar, 84
Witherspoon, John, 54

Wood, George, 141
Woodville, Mississippi, 167–69
Woodward, Joseph, 206–7
Wooster Beach, 158
World Health Organization, 1, 24
Wyman, Walter, 213
Wynkoop, Benjamin, 87

yellow fever: and Black immunity, 22–24; contemporary existence and mortality, 24; etiology and symptoms, 18–20, 27; and European colonization, 20–22, 212; and Spanish American War, 211–16
—, epidemics: in Mobile, Alabama, 160–62; in New Haven, Baltimore, and New York, 84–85; in New Orleans, 164–66, 207–8; in Philadelphia, 3–5, 7–9, 11, 15–18, 26–28, 34–38, 42, 71–84, 85–89; post–Civil War, 207–9; in the South, 164, 208–9; in Woodville, Mississippi, 167–69. *See also* Philadelphia epidemic of 1793
—, mortality: contemporary, 24; in Cuba, 212, 213; in New Orleans, 165; in Philadelphia in 1793, 17–18, 28; in Saint-Domingue, 212; in the South in 1878, 208

www.ingramcontent.com/pod-product-compliance
Lightning Source LLC
Chambersburg PA
CBHW030613230426
43661CB00053B/1962